TABLE OF CONTENTS

TABLE OF CONTENTS

THE PERFORMANCE THERAPIST CERTIFICATION

Master Education Program
Level I Training Manual

EDUCATION VISION

We provide an on-going system of cutting-edge continuing education and development to a network of providers around the world who work to create a fundamental shift in how we think about health and wellness, providing our patients, clients, and customers with a more preventative action approach leading to long-term success.

We take a full, 360° approach to health and wellness that incorporates lifestyle, environmental factors, and the latest research and development, and nurtures the knowledge and intuitive process of the provider and its application so that we get to the root cause of injury and disease and aid in healing from the inside out.

1,000,000

We have a goal. We all got into the health and fitness fields for a reason. We want to make our communities healthier. Our goal is to impact the health and vitality of over 1,000,000 people in the next 5-10 years by taking them out of chronic pain and disease and increasing their ability to perform at a high level. By certifying each of you, we can ALL make a huge difference!

EDUCATION MISSION

LET'S DO THIS TOGETHER!

ABOUT PERFORMANCE THERAPY ACADEMY

Performance Therapy Academy was born out of a desire to bring together all professions that deal with health and vitality. Often, we are sectioned off in our various fields and told that our individual specialties contain the answers to our clients' problems. We begin to believe that, and forget that each of us holds only a piece of the puzzle that makes up our patients' overall wellness. By doing this we fragment the profession and lose sight of the end goal which really is to be a beacon for hope and a deliverer of change for everyone we see.

No doctor, acupuncturist, personal trainer, or wellness coach wants to see diabetes, heart disease, chronic pain, and obesity skyrocket; yet, the health care profession has become broken, overtaken by bottom-line economics and the outcomes of our modern day lifestyles as evidenced by the growing incidences of cancer, childhood obesity, hormone imbalances, early onset diabetes, and more.

Our classes are attended by anyone in the health, fitness, nutrition, and therapy professions looking to increase their personal knowledge and toolsets to better serve their clients as well as other trainers and educators who are a part of the movement that advances these goals. We have a strong belief in collaborating and working together to create amazing outcomes for people who are struggling through the most difficult of health conditions.

Imagine for a moment that you are suffering chronically from pain; you are lethargic all the time with a lack of focus and on the verge of depression and loss of hope. You walk into a health practice or gym and are seeking understanding, compassion, and answers. Two scenarios could occur here. The first is our current system. You wait for between half an hour and one hour in a crowded waiting room; you finally get called back after filling out a mountain of paperwork that briefly asks you your medical history and mostly has you signing insurance and payment forms. You walk into the doctor's office or trainer's sales room and have a 7-10-minute conversation about your situation after which you are either sold on a training package, gym membership and supplements, or a set of labs, procedures, or pills.

Now imagine the future of healthcare. You have highly compassionate and intuitive providers who team up to provide high-level comprehensive care. They spend an hour or two with you learning about your life, your history, and your circumstances. They discuss a plan with you that fits into your current lifestyle while at the same time showing you the path out of the situation you are in and inspiring you again with the possibilities of how this new life would impact you, your children and family, and friends. They offer a protocol tailored to your specific needs, and you walk away with a plan and a support system to execute that plan and keep you on course!

Together, we will do something about it! Together, we will create a movement towards a new way of living and a new way of thinking about health. Together, we educate ourselves, our clients, and our communities to live a new paradigm of Healthy Living. Together, we will make a difference.

WHAT IS YOUR DEFINITION OF A MEDICAL EXERCISE SPECIALIST?

DO YOU HAVE ANY EXPERIENCES IN THIS FIELD? EXPLAIN.

DISCUSSION

REMEMBER !

We help doctors and therapists develop strategic alliances to better your business. We do not take the place of a medical professional under any circumstance.

Remember that as you go through this training and are developing specific training skills, mindset is one of the most important tools. You are not taking an M.D. course or a Physical Therapy Course. You want to provide a service that doctors, PT's, D.C.'s, naturopaths, nutritionists, etc. will gladly refer patients to. Most of the time they have only until insurance runs out to treat a patient and they WANT to find the best people to send them to so that their patients achieve greater outcomes.

There is a reason why DPT's, DO's, and orthopedic surgeons are hesitant to refer patients to personal trainers and people who are solely trained as exercise professionals. The trainer that is louder than the music and motivation is more important than knowing the limits of medical conditions and symptoms. We all have heard of the trainers that will push clients beyond limits. What a trainer may see as weakness of character or will power, a medically-savvy therapist may see as a condition that requires alternate approaches.

We have leaned toward the medical side in this manual to educate trainers and to gain access to these medical professionals. We must be medically proficient in both how we think about and how we look at the body.

If you go after this market, your business can skyrocket and you may not only obtain financial success, you will also gain the respect of your community of colleagues. You will be an important part of the Future of Medicine!!!

There are many ways to grow a business like this. A strategic marketing plan should be in place as you roll out this new way of thinking. You should be considering complementary partners who add to your practice directly. This means you all are in the health and fitness field; however, you each have your own specialty. Next are the partners that you wouldn't normally assume are typical partnerships. You are in the wellness field, but you know of a hairdresser in the area. That hairdresser comes across hundreds of people a week - all of whom talk and complain all day long. You can create a strategic relationship with this hairdresser to refer clients to you.

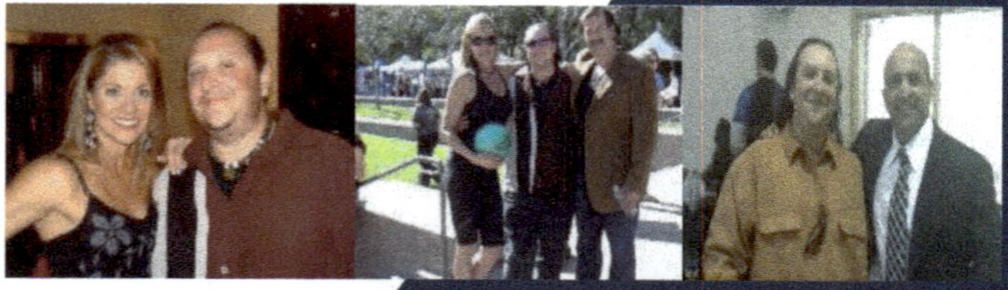

"Everyone has blind spots. Everyone has areas of expertise and areas where they just don't see. The trick is knowing your blind spots and filling themwith the expertise of others."

Ari Gronich, The Performance Therapist

INTERACTIVE BUSINESS DRILL BEFORE WE GET STARTED - ONE OF OUR OBJECTIVES IS TO GROW YOUR BUSINESS SO YOUR SUCCESS CAN HELP MANY!

Before we go into training to become a Performance Therapist, let's discuss what you do in your business now.

WHO ARE YOUR CURRENT COLLABORATIVE PARTNERS IN THE MEDICAL FIELD?

____

____

____

List 10 businesses that you can go to tomorrow and leave with clients coming to you the next day?

1.
2.
3.
4.
5.
6.
7.
8.
9.
10.

NAME SOME BUSINESS PARTNERS YOU CAN COLLABORATE WITH WHO HAVE INFLUENCE ON A LARGE CLIENT LIST.

____

____

____

CUSTOMER SUCCESS

TESTIMONIALS - CHANGING THE WORLD ONE CLIENT AT A TIME

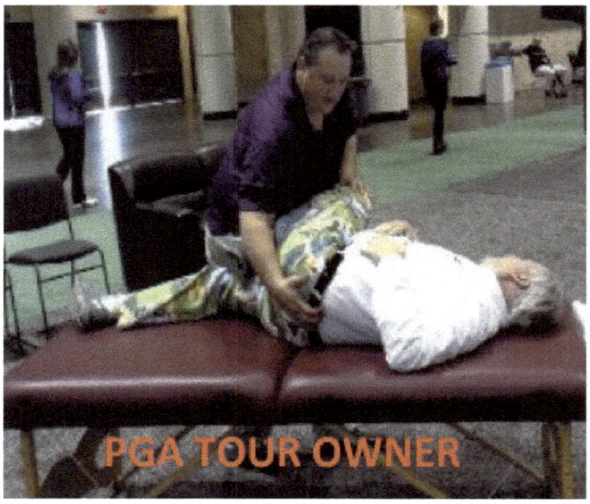

"Hey Ari, I just want to thank you for the advice you've given me while I'm over here in Europe. My leg has gotten increasingly better. This time next year I plan on being just as flexible and strong in my flexibility as you are. Thanks again man. Looking to do more."

Dominique Arnold,
Professional Athlete/110 Meter Hurdler

"Remarkably, because I did not believe it possible considering my condition and history, Ari has taken me farther in my flexibility than I ever expected. Even more remarkably, he has opened up the tightness in both my shoulder and lower back and the total body heaviness and contraction I felt has been replaced with a lightness and ease which makes living in my body a joyful experience once again."

Martin Hannon,
PA-C Physician Assistant

"I have received therapy from Ari Gronich for 3 years, and do not hesitate to recommend him as an extremely skillful therapist."

Neil R. Gumenick,
M.Ac, C.T. L.Ac, Dipl. Ac, Acupuncturist

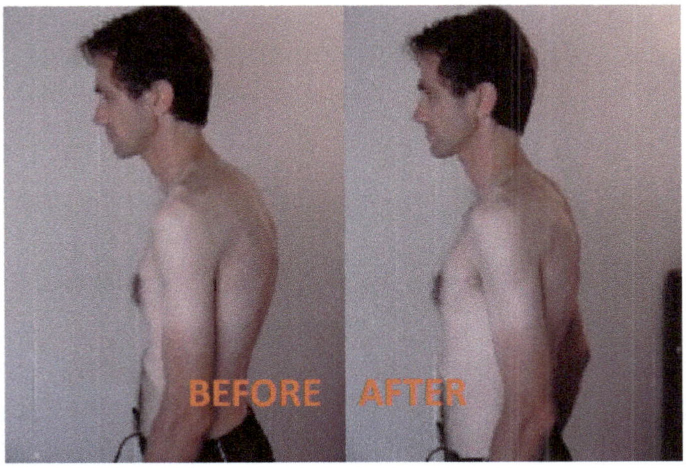

"You have helped me a lot in this past year with being healthy and by showing me how important it is to exercise. You have improved my golf game by 11 strokes and given me a desire to learn more about health. You are a good, knowledgeable, and caring teacher."

Larry Gilmore,
Business Executive

"His comprehensive approach is not "just therapy," but rather an in-depth approach from many disciplines from the physical therapy acumen that rehabilitate the patient in a very efficient and close hands-on format, that has not been seen by me by other facilities that acknowledge their expertise with rehabilitation. Mr. Gronich's approach is totally unique and highly comprehensive; patients will respond much more effectively with this adjunctive intervention."

Michael Szapko,
Chiropractor.

"He has been providing me with back injury and stress management therapy for the last three months. During this time, my back pain in my lower left side has been nearly completely eliminated, my trunk rotation has been greatly expanded, and I can turn my head to see out the rear window of my car for perhaps the first time in my life. With the improved rotation of my torso, I am now even a better golfer. Would you believe my last round improved by 12 strokes?"

Dean Hanley, the Ryan Group,
Marketing Executive

LEGALITIES

Before we get started, let's discuss some of the legalities of working as Performance Therapists

TOUCHING YOUR CLIENTS?

There are different requirements, which vary from state to state, when putting your hands on a client. Make sure that you stay well within these requirements so that your liability is limited and your clients are most at ease. You can find this information by going to your state's regulating website. We highly suggest a disclosure form that is custom-designed for your business. Client should initial each section of the form and sign at the end. If you are not a licensed medical provider, the disclosure form must inform clients that you are NOT a medical doctor or other licensed health care provider. It should also state that any advice and treatment you offer is based on your training and experience and should always be discussed with a doctor or licensed health care professional. There are some states that have a Freedom of Choice policy in the health sector. We are including a few examples of the form and bill for California in the Appendix section of this manual.

LEGAL FORMS AND DISCLAIMERS

Always provide your clients, in the initial intake process and when signing them up as a client, a contract of client rights and responsibilities along with a waiver of liability and terms of dispute resolution. In some cases, there may be an arbitration or jurisdiction clause. We provide a number of sample forms in the Appendix section.

SETTING UP YOUR COMPANY AND PRACTICE TO LIMIT PERSONAL LIABILITY

We highly recommend setting your program and company up to be a membership organization so that every client who joins becomes a member under the guidelines that you set up. This is one way to greatly limit personal liability. Acquire more information in the Performance Therapy Academy back office HUB.

INSURANCE NEEDS

There are a multitude of places to obtain practice insurance. Most of the time your specific organization has deals with insurance companies to provide insurance coverage for you under a group plan at greatly reduced rates. A few suggestions are:

Theinsuranceguy.com - Ken Renig is a recommended resource by Achieve Systems.

Massageliabilityinsurancegroup.com - has great rates and covers over 350 modalities of bodywork, kinesiology, etc.

There are many sources to choose from. Shop around and choose the right one for you and your specific field of expertise.

INCIDENT REPORTING

In the Forms Appendix in this manual, find an incident report that you will send to your insurance if there is ever an issue.

WAIVER OF LIABILITY

Always have your clients fill out a liability waiver. We have included one in the Forms Appendix of this manual.

OTHER

To remove personal liability, we would highly recommend setting your company up to protect you. That includes the structure of your company whether you choose to become a C or S corporation or LLC.

The tax structure that you set up will provide greater detail on your protections. Talk with your accountant or financial adviser. We use www.amerilawyer.com. They can set up the corporation and act as your Registered Agent. The Registered Agent yearly fee includes a free General Counsel Club that answers any legal questions any time day or night. They will listen to your needs and provide you with the added benefit of being covered by a law firm.

RECOMMENDED SUCCESS TOOLS

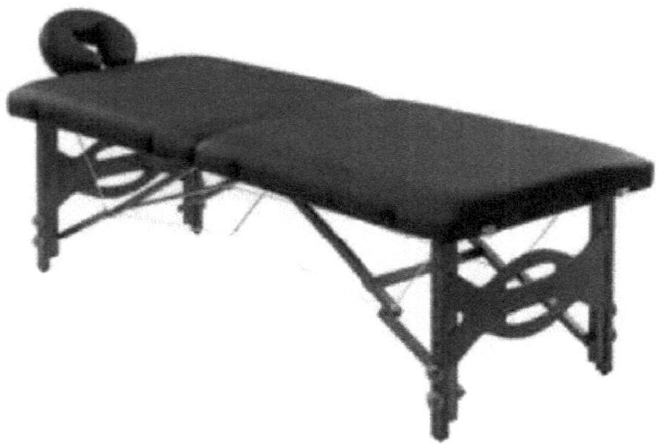

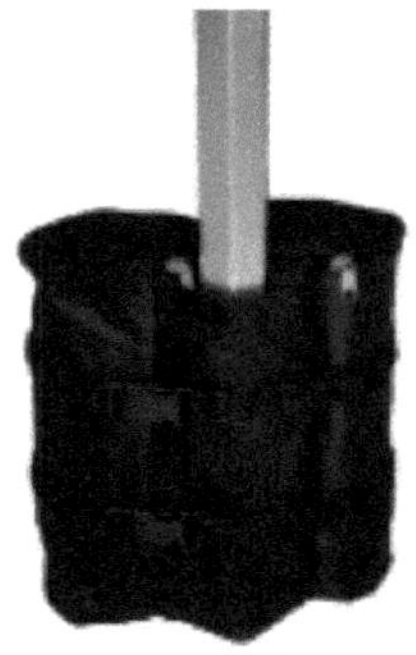

We recommend that every Performance Therapist has his/her own table to use for working on clients and evaluating them. We also recommend weighted table leg bags if you have a portable lightweight table. These will be invaluable to stabilize the table and keep it from falling over during specific exercise movements. Look at the attached exhibit for power partners if you do not have a table.

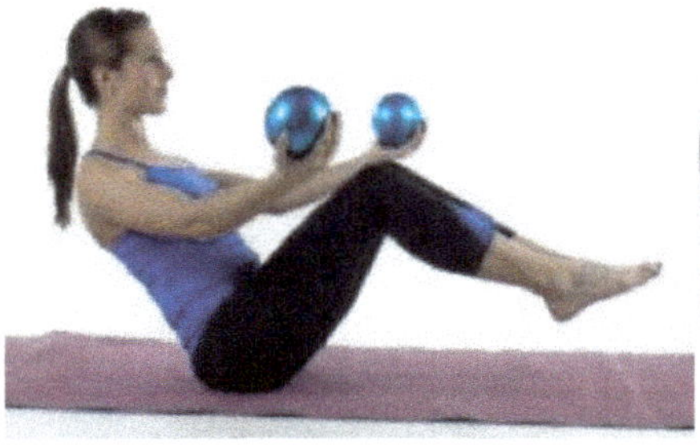

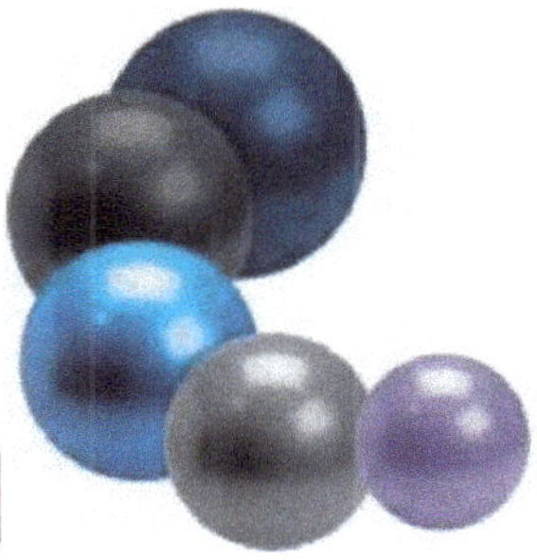

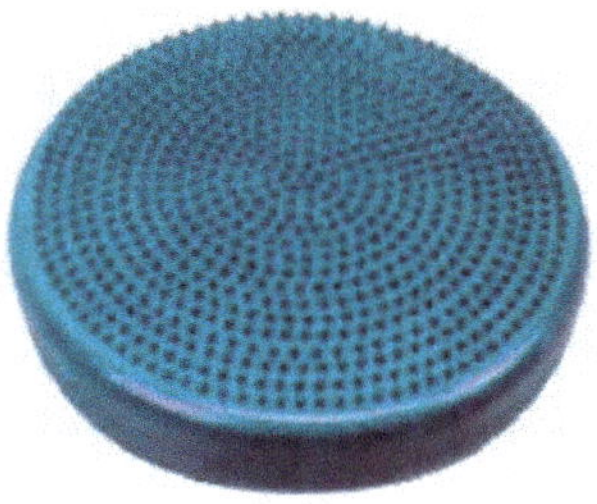

Weighted yoga balls, sized exercise balls, and exercise discs will also provide practitioners with great resources for resistance and positional training. They cause imbalances that force clients' bodies to compensate and therefore help build strength and balance in the body.

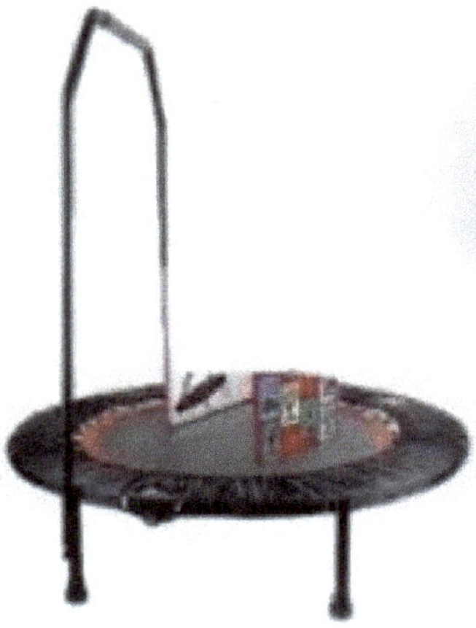

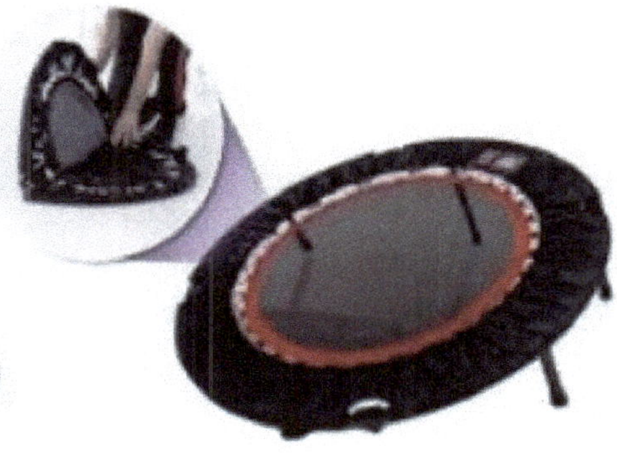

A rebounder is good for many situations. You can train for balance, lymphatic drainage and detoxification of the lymph system, oxygenation of cells, and drawing nutrients out of the blood and into the muscles. It is one of the best tools for rebuilding bone growth, especially for those with osteoporosis. It is even great for training muscle cell endurance.

LEVEL I
PERFORMANCE THERAPIST CERTIFICATE: WHAT YOU WILL LEARN TODAY

MODULE I
DURATION: 3 HOURS

Introduction to Developing Your Intuition and Evaluation Skills

Learning the basics of palpation and honing your senses to be able to know and understand a client's needs.

During Module I you will be guided through hands-on experiences in a series of exercises that will enhance your diagnostic prowess and enable you to provide your clients with the highest level of individualized care. Rather than relying on general knowledge alone, you will begin enhancing your senses and sensitivities in order to better understand your clients. With your heightened awareness, you will have the ability to work with clients from all walks of life and with a broad spectrum of ailments, providing them with a unique service that they can only get from YOU!

MODULE II
DURATION: 2 HOURS

Introduction to Multi-Directional Resistance Stretching© - Lower Body

In the fitness world, there are many opinions when it comes to stretching. For some, flexibility training gets a bad rap and is deemed to be counterproductive to high performance. Some of the people in our industry hold the concept that not stretching before major exertion in sports is a good idea. The old school ways we were taught to stretch as kids can cause injuries and damage. We all remember trying to reach our toes and bouncing up and down to attempt a deeper stretch. Archaic stretching techniques can be boring, tedious, and take a long time to see results, so why do them?

This introductory course will awaken you to the new possibilities of flexibility training. Beginning from the ground up, we will experience the opening of our feet, ankles, calves, and knees, continuing all the way up through the lower half of our body into the hips and pelvis and the lower core muscles.

The majority of injury and pain in our bodies is due to stiff muscles that are not prepared for the movements we call on them to perform. Flexibility training is not just for sports and athletics. It is also for everyone who wants to prevent or avoid injury caused by slips and falls, trips and flips on stairs, or wet surfaces that cause us to suddenly do the splits. It is essential for just walking from the parking lot and through a store for an hour.

Tumbling down stairs is the number one reason people wind up in the ER, according to data from the **National Electronic Injury Surveillance System** (NEISS) which is maintained by the U.S. Consumer Product Safety Commission. In 2014, there were an estimated 1.14 million visits to U.S. emergency rooms in which steps or stairs played a role in the injury. The second reason people wind up in the ER is slipping and falling due to wet surfaces on the floor.

Help your clients avoid the ER by providing them with a prepared flexible lower body.

MODULE III
DURATION: 2 HOURS

Introduction to Multi-Directional Resistance Stretching© - Upper Body

In this module we continue from the lower body to the upper body, beginning at the upper pelvic center of the core and continuing to the lower abdomen, rib cage, upper abdomen, and throughout the muscles of the back, shoulders, neck, and arms.

With increased flexibility comes an increase in leverage, and with an increase in leverage comes a greater amount of power and strength. This allows us to perform at peak levels with all sports as well as help avoid injury and pain in our most vulnerable areas such as lumbar spine, cervical spine, and shoulders.

Far too many people have difficulty with everyday tasks such as bending and lifting, raising their arms over their heads, and more. We have all heard patients and clients come to us and say, "Doc said I might get back to 80%," or "the trainer told me I would never be as good as I was!"

This introduction to the upper body will give you a winning edge when working with new clients and patients. You will get them out of injury faster, help them heal more completely, and put them back into the world better than you found them.

LEVEL I: MODULE I

DEVELOPING YOUR INTUITION AND EVALUATION SKILLS

MODULE I: DEVELOPING YOUR INTUITION AND EVALUATION SKILLS

Most of you in this room have years of experience running clients through functional tests that give you a baseline of where someone is - GAIT testing, plank testing for balance and core strength, etc. If you are a PT or DC, you have X-rays and MRI's as well as a multitude of other tools that can give insight into a client's structure. Doctors and nutritionists have relied on blood tests and clinically-designed questionnaires that can give a general basis for understanding clinical conditions and lifestyle behavior patterns.

It is important that when we begin working together for the common good of our clients, we begin to educate ourselves on each other's protocols. For too many years we have either dismissed the work our colleagues do as ineffective or inferior to our own. In some cases, we have simply remained completely uneducated on what each other does. This makes it very difficult to both give and receive referrals from each other and provide high level results for our clients.

(Helpful Hint): "It is much easier to get a doctor to send you referrals when you make them a client! Healthy doctors equal healthy patients."

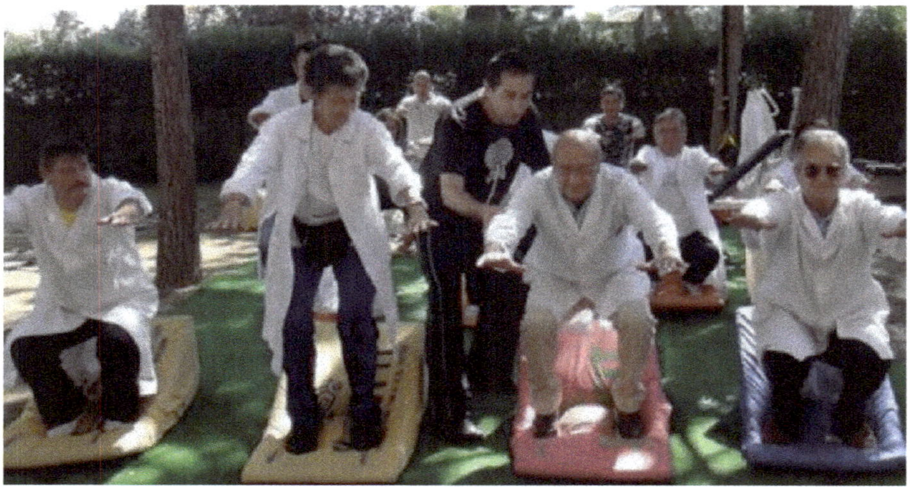

http://www.slowfit.com/en/images/schede/59gallery2.jpg

For many in the profession, due to liabilities, insurance rules, and a change in the dynamics of scope of practice, we have gotten away from the basics of intuitive medicine and evaluation. Shamans and medicine men used to travel to the homes of their patients and, in some cases, stay awhile in order to get an overall sense of the lifestyle their clients were living. That kind of in-depth medicine has all but died out, leaving a health practitioner to rely on a limited amount of information as well as limited time for diagnoses.

> *"Our outcomes have suffered from the inability to truly spend time getting to know our clients. We must find other ways to tune in to our senses and use our vast tools to make up for this new way of living."*
>
> **Ari Gronich, The Performance Therapist**

As a student, I had a blind massage therapist who taught us the value of listening, smelling, and feeling with our fingers what was happening with a client. He would blindfold us in class so that we could get attuned to our other senses.

Another was a master of functional anatomy and kinesiology who used to say, "You must see with your hands what your eyes cannot see." Because of these two mentors, we begin teaching the start of every class blindfolded.

BLINDFOLD EVALUATION PROCESS

Split up into teams of two. One of you will be client and one practitioner.

Place client on a treatment table.

Place blindfold on or close practitioner's eyes.

INTERACTIVE ASSESSMENT DRILL

CLIENT PRONE (LYING FACE DOWN)

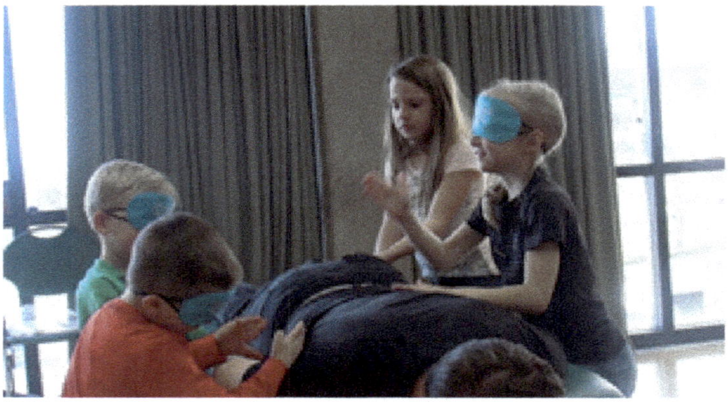

Run your hands along client's feet: first the soles of the feet and then up to the heels and around the ankles. Feel the skin and deeper into the muscles. Feel for muscles that are tight or loose or knotted or smooth. Feel for temperature - hot and cold. Feel if the muscle is having any micro twitches or if it is still.

Move your hands from the ankle to the base of the calves. Push with your thumbs and try to trace the edges of the calf muscles. See with your hands what your eyes cannot see. Feel the direction that the muscle fibers go and again feel for tension spots and soft spots. Feel for weaker muscle and stronger muscle, heat and cold; feel how the muscles respond to your touch.

Do they twitch or have a strong pulse?

Is the person relaxing with your touch or tensing up?

What is happening around you...?

Do you smell anything unusual?

When you shut off one sense, it empowers and enlivens the others. Is your hearing becoming more acute?

What do you hear happening under your fingers?

Can you hear and feel the breathing patterns of your client?

WHAT'S NEXT...

Now your intuition is beginning to build

Where do your hands want to take you next?

Do they want you to continue in the pattern of going directly up the body or are your hands being called to another part of the body?

Maybe you are hearing a voice in your subconscious telling you to connect two areas of the body or jump to another part of the body altogether.

You are feeling muscles and bones and ligaments and tendons and veins and lymph nodes.

Can you sense and imagine everything you are touching is reacting to you and communicating with you in some way, telling you what is happening with this person?

As your hands glide across the glutes and your thumbs and fingers dig a little deeper into the various muscles, they can feel if there is a jump or reflex in the muscle, and which side is higher or lower. Feel if the hips and pelvic bone are even or do they feel twisted and turned? It is amazing how clear the senses are getting in your fingers. They are growing in sensitivity and feeling every nuance.

Continue this movement all the way up to the back being sure to feel for lymph nodes and whether the back is straight or twisted, hot or cold, knotty or smooth. Feel for the ribcage and the space in between each rib for mobility and flexibility; feel all of the muscles and the different directions they go up the entire back.

Is the tension the same on both sides?

Does the spine feel high or low on either side?

Are there any areas where the spine is not in a straight line as you drift your thumbs from the sacrum to the base of the skull?

As your hands are sensing, you are reminding your brain to remember the areas you are feeling and what you are feeling because you will be marking this information down on a client sheet. This will allow you to have a progress report that your client can look at between sessions. It will definitely help them see results even when they may not be feeling them, and it is a good way to document the imbalances and balances your client is having. You may even be able to tie these results to what was happening in between sessions on an emotional, physical, or stress-level scale.

DISCUSSION & NOTES:

INTERACTIVE DRILL

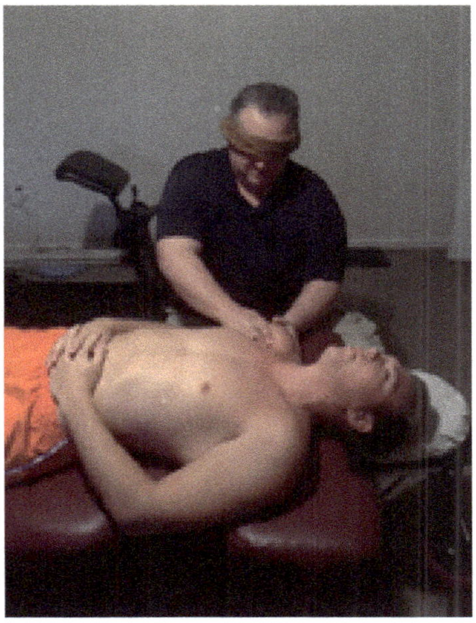

CLIENT SUPINE (LYING FACE UP)

Again, begin at the feet. Feel how tense and tight or loose and flexible the toes and tops of the feet are. Move around the foot while holding the base of the foot and ankle and get an idea of how much range of motion is there.

Does the joint grind?

Does it pop and adjust into place, or is it stiff and immobile?

Do the feet want to lie flat on the heel, or do they tend to go out to the sides or in towards the centerline?

Depending on which way they are going, you may note either a weakness or a tightness in the hips' adductors and abductors.

Glide your thumbs up the edge of the tibia and tibialis muscle gently noticing if the muscle is elastic or taut, again also feeling for heat or cool, smooth or knotted. Make sure you are gliding along the entire upper portion of the leg to find scar tissue, weaknesses, and strengths.

Feel the knee joint.

Is there swelling or scar tissue? Does the knee feel stable or imbalanced?

Grab underneath the knee joint and lift the leg, bending the knee to get a sense of range of motion. Listen to the hip as you lift the leg.

Is the person tightening up or allowing for the movement and motion?

As you move up the body with your hands, you will also be moving up the sides of the table. For this portion either side is okay to go up first; just make sure you get to both sides of the body.

If a person is tensing up through this motion even though the ligaments and tendons feel loose, then that person may be uncomfortable with the movement. This may be an underlying sign of how he or she handles being out of their comfort zone and something you could help with as you train and rehabilitate them. Hesitancy and mistrust may be there as well, so just pay attention to the signs that you cannot see.

Glide your hands up towards the hip bones and feel if they are twisted up or down, in or out, high or low. Note in your mind which side feels tenser and which is more relaxed.

Now we are going to move up into the abdominals feeling for tension, smoothness, temperature, etc. Move up into the rib cage checking for flexibility and for breathing.

"Remember that you are a medical exercise professional. Your doctor is not shy about seeing you naked or working with problem areas on your body. Why then should you be uncomfortable with your clients? Be respectful of your client's body; however, this should not be to the detriment of their health. Getting permission ahead of time with boundaries is necessary and professional. The more comfortable YOU are knowing what you are doing and that you are doing what is most beneficial for their overall health, the more comfortable your client will be with whatever you are doing for them."

Ari Gronich, The Performance Therapist

What do you feel? Lumpy or smooth?

Is the client tense or relaxed? Are you?

From here we move to the shoulders - feeling whether the shoulders tend to lay back or curve up.

Is one higher than the other, or tighter than the other?

As you move into the muscles of the neck, you can move the head from side to side to feel for range of motion or tension and lack of movement.

We finish our blind evaluation by simply gliding our fingers from the back of the neck up the occiput, and off of the skull having not only given our client a great warming and relaxing experience, but also having given ourselves a deeper understanding of what is happening in their body. This is imperative to proper training with an eye for injury prevention and performance therapy!

USING THE EVALUATION FORM

When you are finished with each side of your client, mark down on the evaluation form what you noticed. This way you are not relying on memory and you maintain a consistent chart of progress as sessions continue. If you are lucky enough to have a staff member, use that staff member to mark the sheet as you go and dictate directly as you are palpating the body. The more accurate and descriptive, the better.

SWITCH

Now have practitioner and client switch roles and repeat the processes.

DISCUSSION & NOTES:

PALPATION EVALUATION FORM

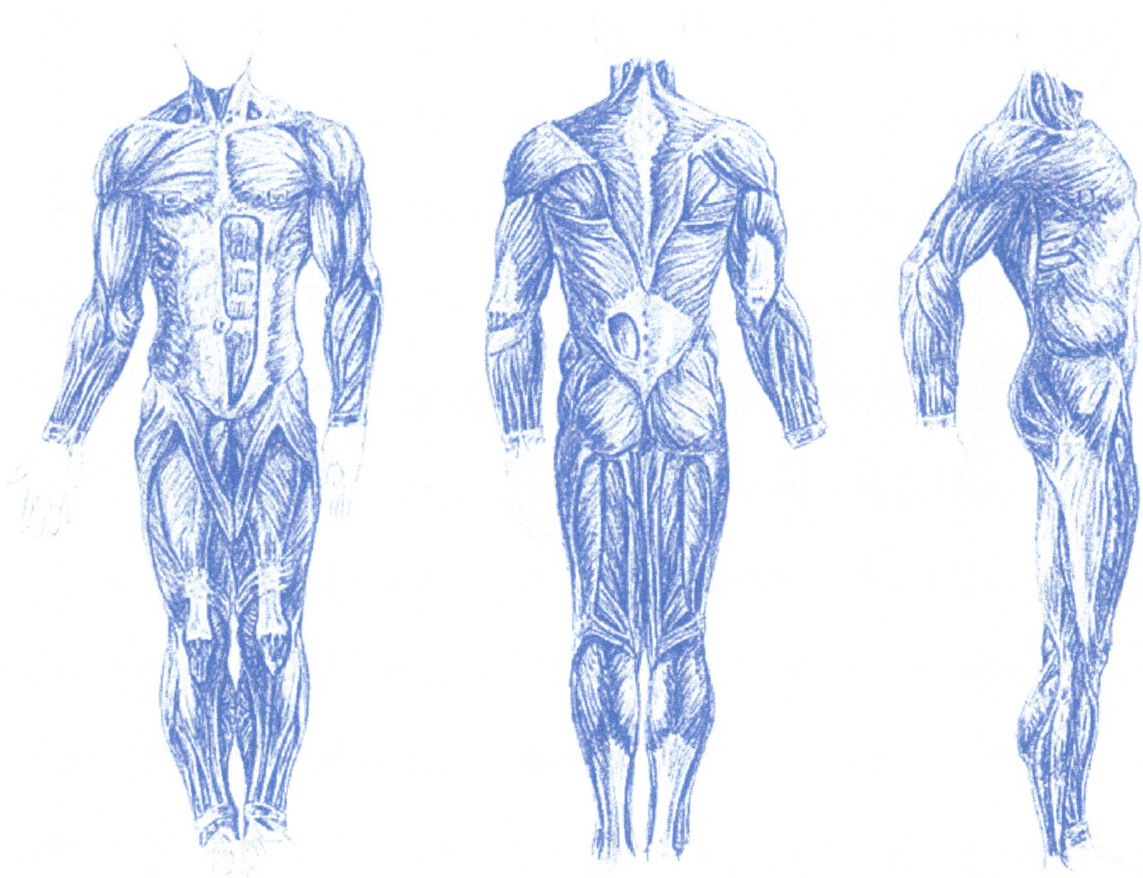

Drawings by: Arvalis

GLOSSARY OF TERMS:

H – HOT	T – TIGHT
C – COLD	R – RELAXED
E – EVEN	TW – TWISTED
SM – SMOOTH	KN – KNOTTED
HIGH – RAISED OR ELEVATED	LOW – SUNKEN OR DEPRESSED
DIRECTION OF TENSION	DIRECTION OF TENSION
P – PULSE	JMP – JUMP REFLEX
GR – GRINDING	LROM – LIMITED RANGE OF MOTION
FRONT OF THE BODY NOTES:	**BACK OF THE BODY NOTES:**

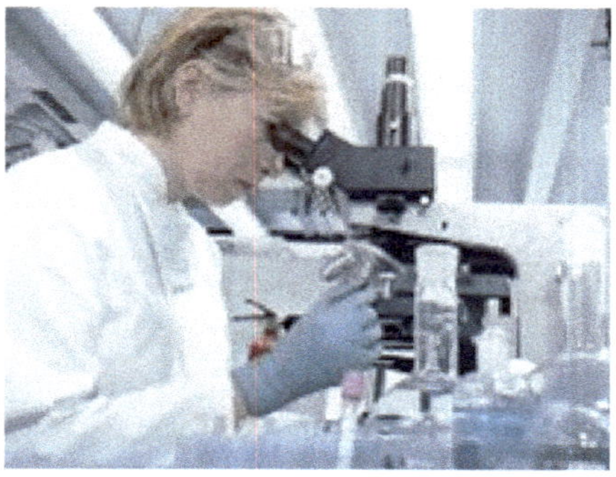

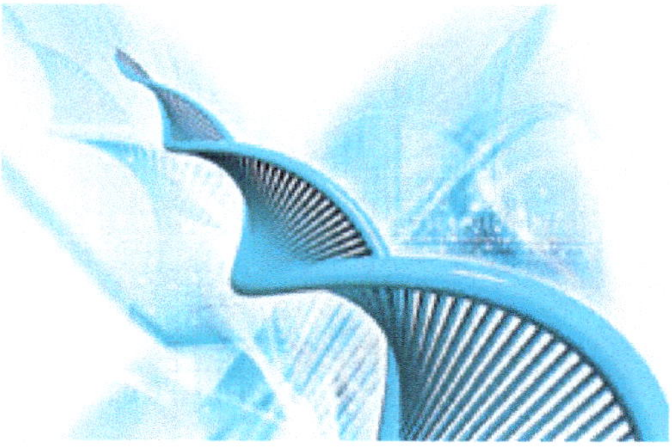

PATHOLOGICAL LAB RANGE VS. FUNCTIONAL LAB RANGE

Lab test results always come back with a range of what is acceptable. This introduction to reading lab test results will instruct you to begin looking at a client's tests with an eye for optimization rather than through the standard range that a majority of the western medical community looks at.

QUESTIONS SECTION

Why do Functional lab ranges differ from Pathological lab ranges?

When we go to the doctor's office and they take our blood and do labs, the results they get can be misleading. According to the book "Blood Chemistry and CBC Analysis" by Dicken Weatherby and Scott Ferguson, pathological ranges are determined by taking a bell curve of 95% of the population deeming them healthy or what is within "Normal" range. If you are on the outsides of those ranges, it means you are already in some level of disease or illness.

Do you believe that 95% of the population is healthy?

Do you believe that if your numbers are within the "average" range that YOU are healthy?

Why could it be that so many people who go to the doctor and get tested for symptoms come up with lab ranges that are within the average pathological range and are told that nothing is wrong with them, even though they are still experiencing symptoms?

How many of you or your clients have gone to a traditional doctor and have been told that your symptoms are in your head and that according to the tests, you are healthy?

Functional Lab ranges are determined by what would be an optimal scenario. For example, if your pathological range for blood glucose is 65 – 110, your doctor would say that you are in a normal range. Functional range for blood glucose is 85 – 100 which would be in the optimal range for functional health. What happens with the in between? Well, if a Functional medicine practitioner is looking at the numbers and your range is between the 65 - 85 or the 100 -110, it may indicate to that practitioner that you have insulin resistance or beginning tendencies towards diabetes or hypoglycemia. These are conditions that could be addressed if you know how to look at the labs and interpret them

This knowledge can be very helpful for a nutritionist or personal trainer when working with a client coming in for weight loss and to ease symptoms of disease and illness. When you are armed with this kind of knowledge, the protocols you develop will shift to get more optimum results - thus increasing your effectiveness and value to your clients.

INTERACTIVE DRILL

IMBALANCE

How would you train someone differently or prescribe a diet differently for someone with a hormonal imbalance, or someone with diabetes, or cholesterol issues?

By beginning to gain knowledge in using the functional range for labs, we can address our clients and patients as a whole being. Rather than just look at health as the absence of disease, we look at health as living an optimum life with plenty of energy during the day, healthy restful sleep at night, and a digestive system that works in proper elimination of toxins and is free from symptomatic issues that lessen our ability to live a quality life.

What things do you look at in the test report to determine wellness?

Once a blood test is completed, we look for what we call "biomarkers" to health, such as:

- Anemia (a lack of iron or B-12)
- Too much iron
- Thyroid problems
- Hidden chronic infections (viral, fungal, or bacterial)
- Adrenal problems
- Digestive problems
- Allergies
- Blood sugar problems
- Liver/gallbladder disorder
- Cardiovascular disorder
- Stroke markers

Dorland's Medical Dictionary defines health as: "A state of optimal physical, mental, and social well-being, and not merely the absence of disease and infirmity."

PATHOLOGICAL VS FUNCTIONAL LAB FORM

Markers	Pathological Range	Functional Range
Glucose	65-110 mg/dl	85-100 mg/dl
Cholesterol	<200 mg/dl	150-200 mg/dl
Triglycerides	<150 mg/dl	75-100 mg/dl
LDL	<130 mg/dl	<120 mg/dl
HDL	>40 mg/dl	>55 mg/dl
Chol/HDL Ratio	<3.7	<3.1
Iron	40-180 ug/dl	85-130 ug/dl
TIBC	250-390 ug/dl	250-350 ug/dl
Ferritin	33-236	(F premenopause) 10-122
	33-236	(F postmenopause) 10-263
		(M) 33-263 ng/ml
Hgb	12-16 grams/dl	(F) 13.5-14.5 (M)14-15
Hct	36-48.2%	(F) 37-44 (M)40-48
RBC	3.9-5.10	(F) 3.9-4.5 (M)4.2-4.9
MCV	82-103 cu microns	85-92 cu microns
MCH	27-34 g/cu microns	27-32 cu microns
MCHC	30.9-35.4 g/cu micron	32-35%
RDW	10.8-14.8 %	<13
Platelets	150,000-400,000	150,000-450,000
WBC	4,000-10,000	5,000-8,000
Neutrophils	40-78%	40-60%
Lymphocytes	15-50%	25-40%
Monocytes	0-13%	<7%
Eosinophils	0-5%	<3%
Basophils	0-5%	0-1%
TSH	0.3-5.7mlU/L	1.8-3.0 mlU/L
T4	4.5-12.5 mg/dl	6-12 mg/dL
T3 Uptake	27-37 %	28-38 %
FTI	4.6-10.9 mg/dl	6-11 index units
SGOT (AST)	1/45 U/L	10-26 U/L
SGPT (ALT)	1/55 U/L	10-26 U/L
GGTP	5-52U/L	10-26 U/L
LDH	89-215 U/L	140-180 U/L
Alk. Phos.	27-142 U/L	70-90 U/L
Total Bilirubin	0.1-1.5 mg/dl	0.2-1.2 mg/dl
Total Protein	6.2-8.3 G/dl	6.9-7.4 G/dl
Albumin	3.8-5.0 G/dl	4.0-5.0 G/dL
Globulin	2.0-3.8 G/100 ml	2.4-2.8 G/100mL
A/G Ratio	1.1-2.3 units	1.5-2.0 units
Sodium	135-148 mmol/L	135-140 mmol/L

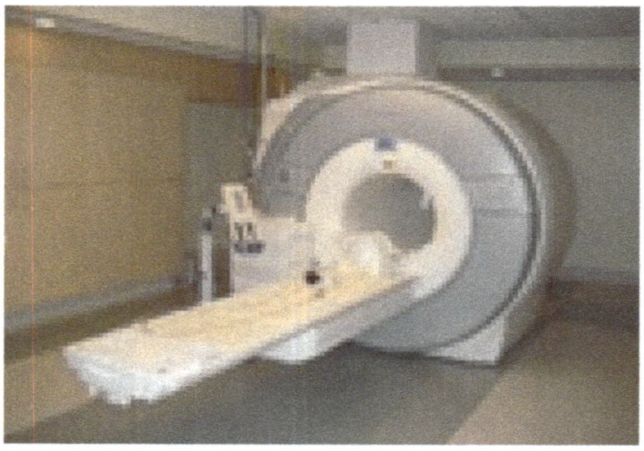

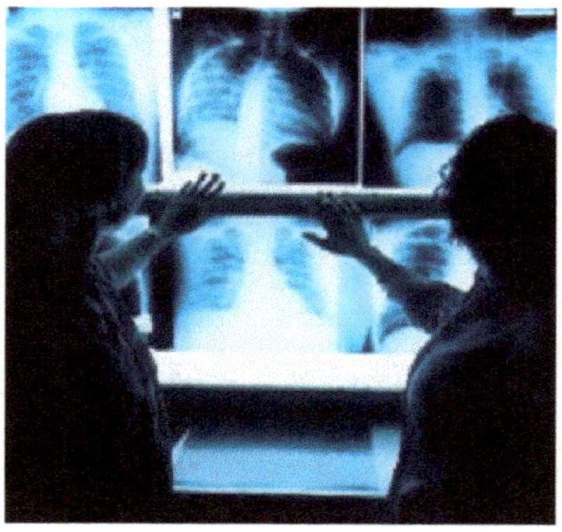

X-RAYS AND MRI'S

Let's Learn How to Evaluate to Help Your Clients!

A GREAT TOOL FOR MEDICAL FITNESS AND ALTERNATIVE HEALTH PROFESSIONALS TO LEARN

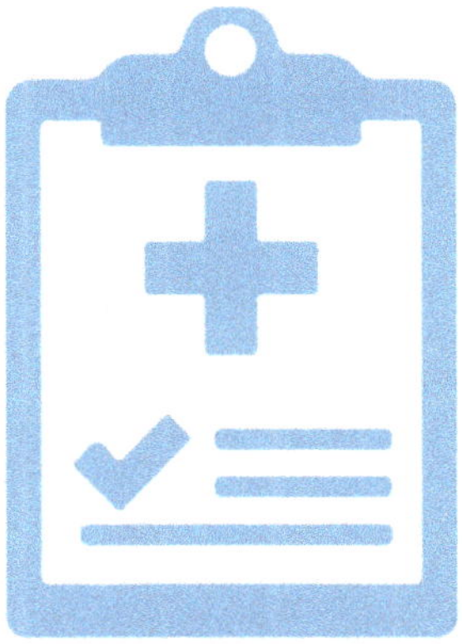

X-rays and MRI's are great diagnostic tools for evaluation as well. However, reading the reports for content is different from reading the images. When you can look into a body, you can gain a deeper understanding of how to apply your therapy or training to optimize the experience and not only aid in the prevention of injury but help to quickly rehabilitate someone so they become better than they were before.

When we learn to read the images of a spine, we can find injury which will enable us to avoid over training as well as understand areas that need strengthening. Unless you are a chiropractor or medical doctor, it is not within your scope of practice to diagnose from these images; however, if you can look at the report and look at the images, remember what you felt when scanning the body blindfolded, and call upon your knowledge of anatomy and physiology. All together, you will have a greater sense of knowing what is happening within that client who is in front of you.

"Asking for X-ray and MRI results should be commonplace for a great Performance Therapist so you show your professionalism and competency which will lead to strong branding for your practice!"

Ari Gronich, The Performance Therapist

INTERACTIVE DRILL

IMAGE TRAINING

Let's review some of the images below so that you can get a basic understanding of what you are looking at as well as how what you see in the images translates to what you feel when you are palpating the body.

When you get to the next level and we include shoulder girdles, rotator cuffs, bicep tendons and joints, ankles, knees, etc., you will have a greater insight into what is happening in your clients. With this deep understanding of the human frame, anatomy, kinesiology, and the nervous system, you will be armed with the functional knowledge of how to use your skills to achieve the highest quality results, and you may prevent future injuries from occurring.

Do you have any experiences in reading images?

DISCUSSION & NOTES:

What are physical signs you can see without an MRI which show that a person has Degenerative Disc Disease?

When a client comes to you with loss of flexibility, weakness and tingling or numbness in legs, or possible bowel and bladder control issues, these may be signs of Degenerative Disc Disease.

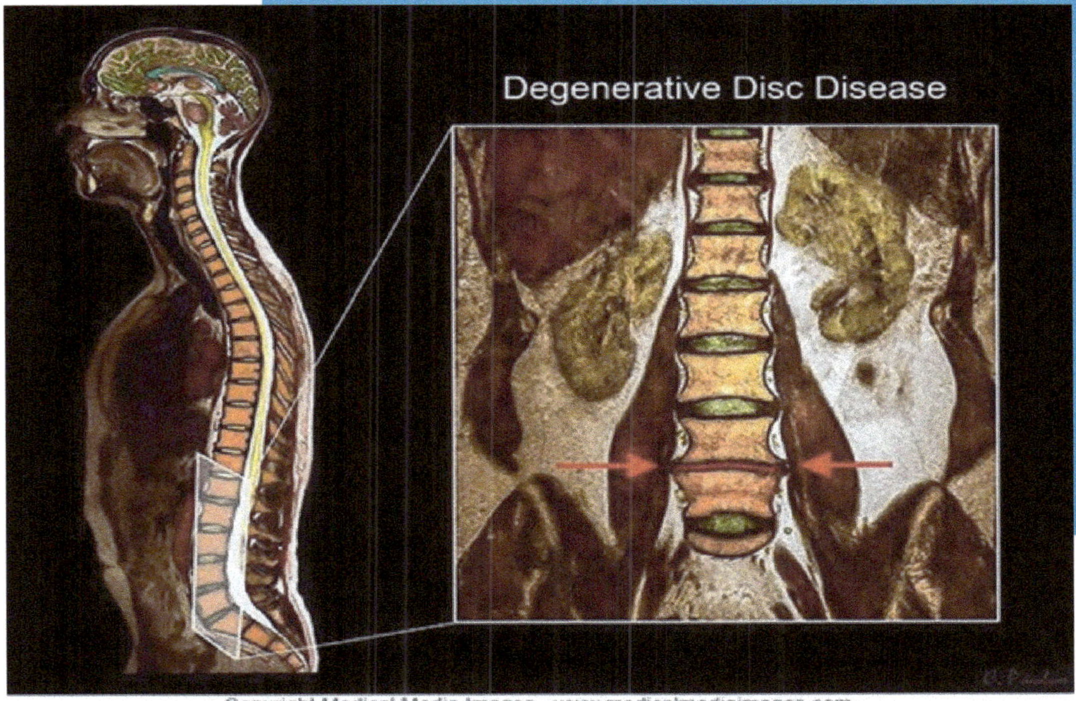

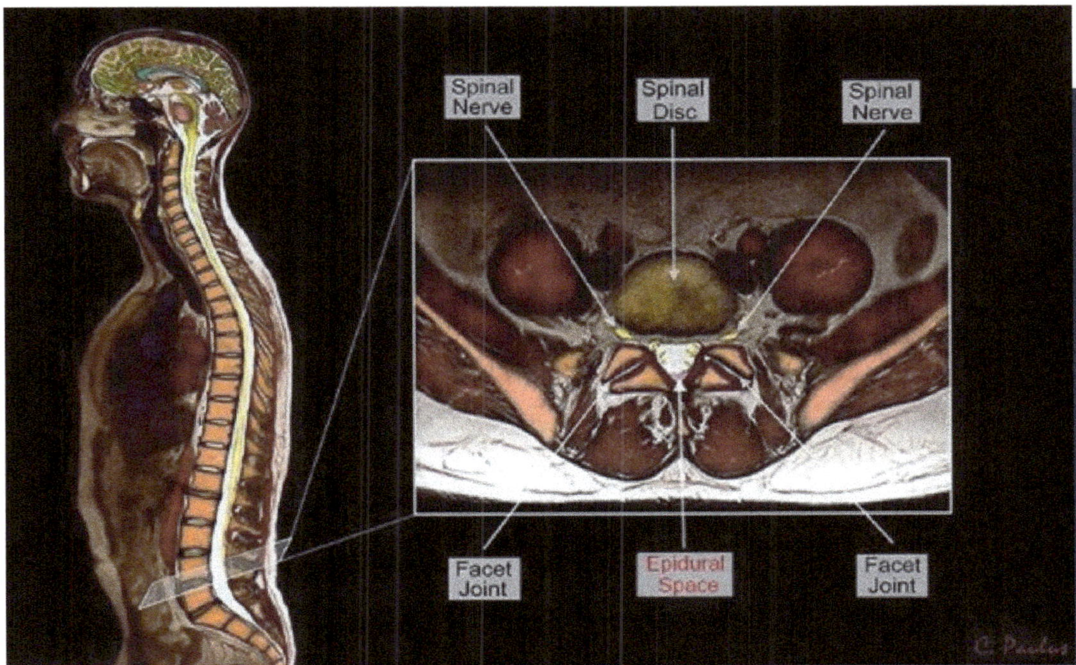

Bending, lifting, and twisting may make pain worse in patients with Degenerative Disc Disease. When creating an exercise program, make sure the movements are slow and methodical to avoid exacerbating this disease!

Narrowing of the epidural space can be caused by steroid epidurals or even obesity. This can cause neurological problems and radicular symptoms such as leg pain, numbness, and tingling including symptoms of sciatica.

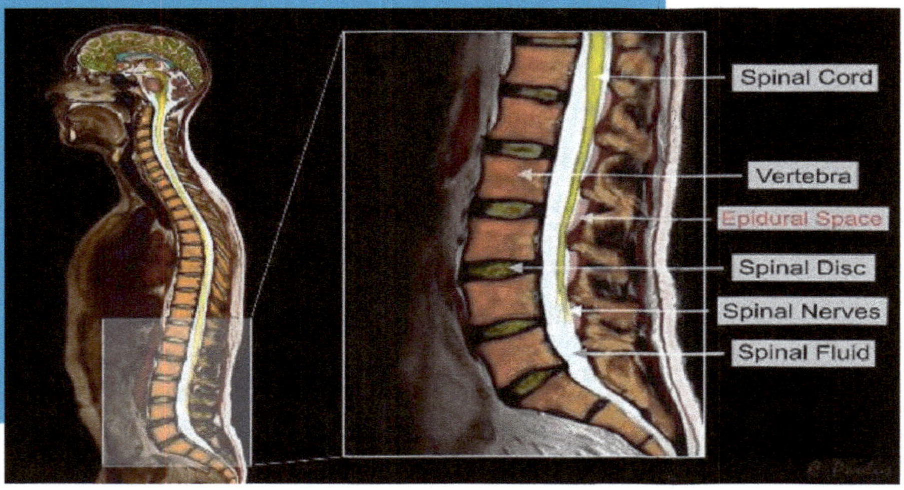

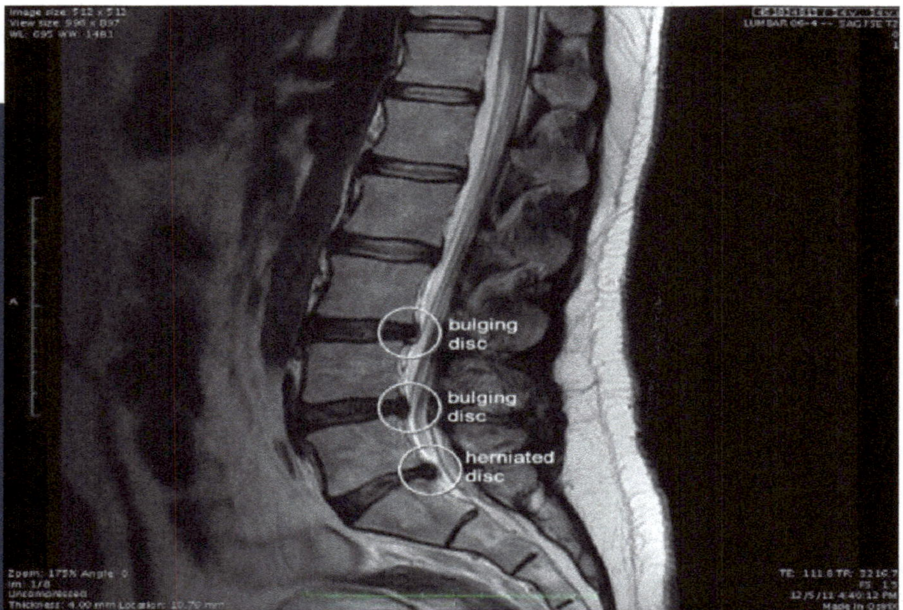

Regardless of what you may have heard, bulging and herniated discs do not have to be permanent injuries. Exercises must be designed to allow our muscles to support the low back without triggering more pain or causing further injury. The traditional knee to chest exercise is an example of what NOT to do.

EXERCISE TO HELP

Lengthening the abdominal muscles and psoas while contracting, tightening, and supporting the lumbar muscles will trigger the body to support and heal those discs in a more expedient way as well as cause less damage and pain to your patient.

Take an exercise ball and place it between the glutes and ankles of your client. Have them lean back slightly, stretching the abdominal muscles, then squeeze the ball between the glutes and ankles. This will engage the entire core muscle group. Place your hands on the client's shoulder blades as a spotter for this movement and help motivate them to squeeze until fatigued. At that point gently spot them back to a neutral position before doing the movement again. It is important to have a spotter take them through the ROM in this exercise so that upon returning to the neutral position they do not overstrain the lumbar muscles.

As you can see in the pictures below, you are guiding the client into a position where they are almost lying on the ball. However, from this position they are squeezing the ball from ankles towards glutes and mostly holding up their own body weight thus activating all of the abdominal muscles. This strengthens the entire musculature aiding in the healing and supporting of the low back and herniated or bulging discs.

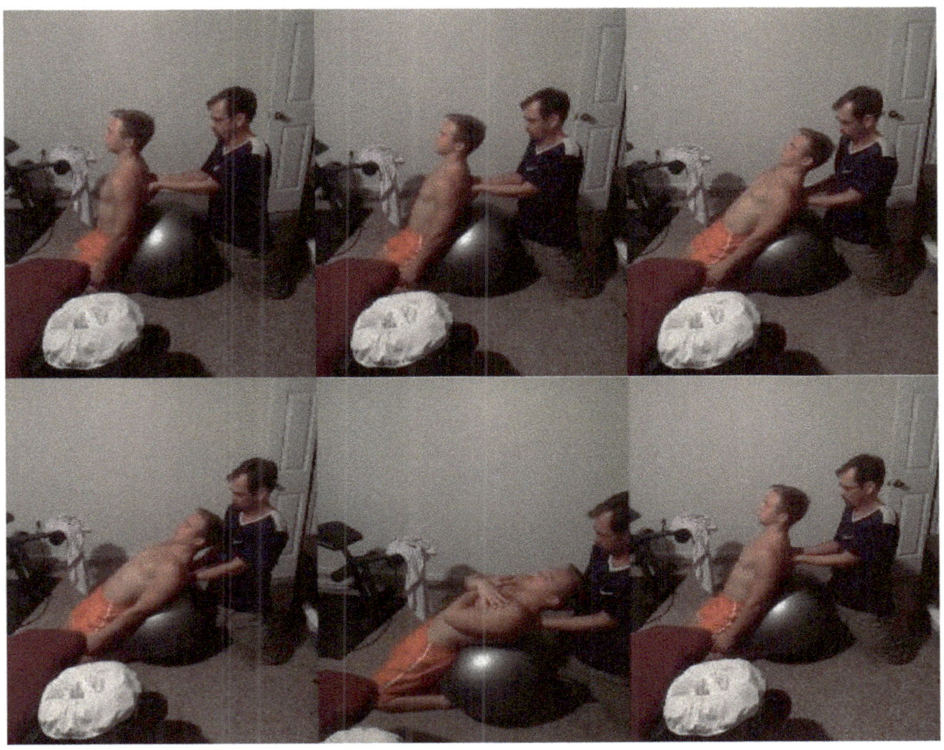

Cervical Spinal Stenosis is more rare and dangerous than lumbar stenosis. With cervical stenosis, symptoms can lead to coordination issues beyond the normal pain. With lumbar stenosis, sciatica symptoms are more common. Exercises for ROM are important as well as slow steady movement. Tai Chi, light swimming and water therapy, non intense yoga, as well as MDRS (Multi-Directional Resistance Stretching) are helpful for treating lumbar stenosis.

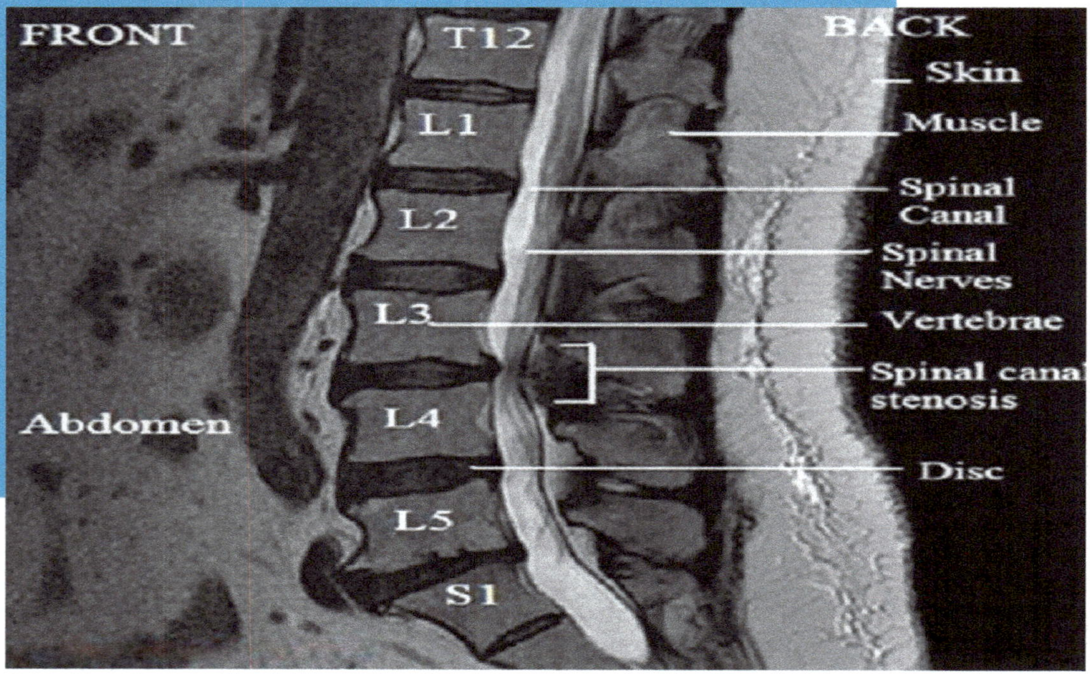

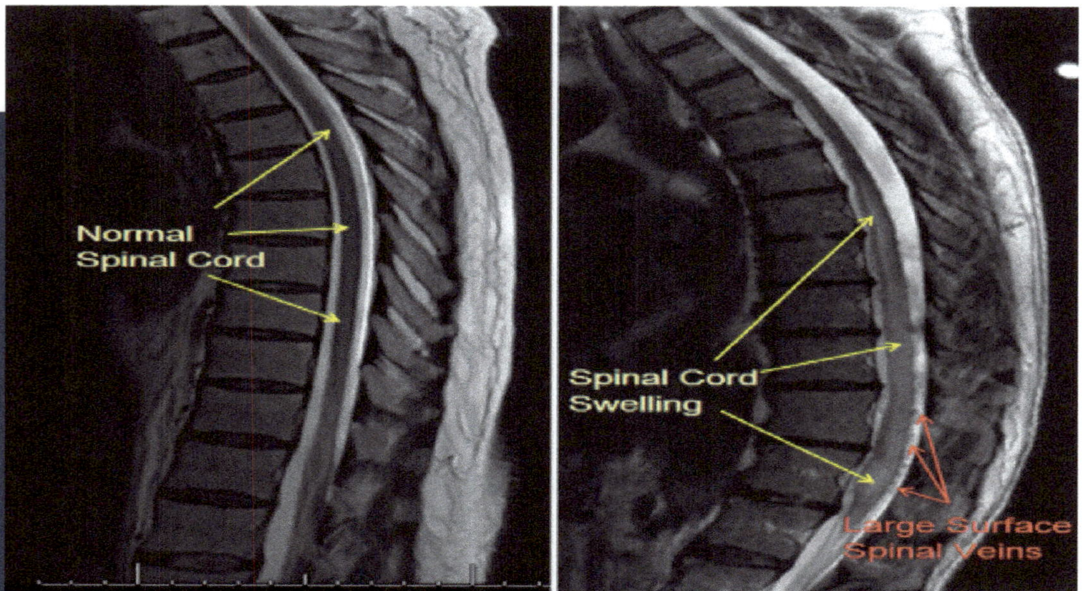

Injuries that cause swelling are typical from intense twisting trauma that occurs with car accidents or improper exercises. Even chiropractic adjustments that target the lumbar spine in a twisting action can be delivered hard enough to cause swelling in the spinal cord.

When this occurs, manual traction on an inversion table can be very helpful. Place your client on the inversion table at a 60 degree angle so they are only slightly upside down. Then place your hands under the shoulder blades, gently lifting them up off the table. Slowly move them from side to side allowing their body to gently decompress in the spine and allowing space to grow and take pressure off of the spinal cord.

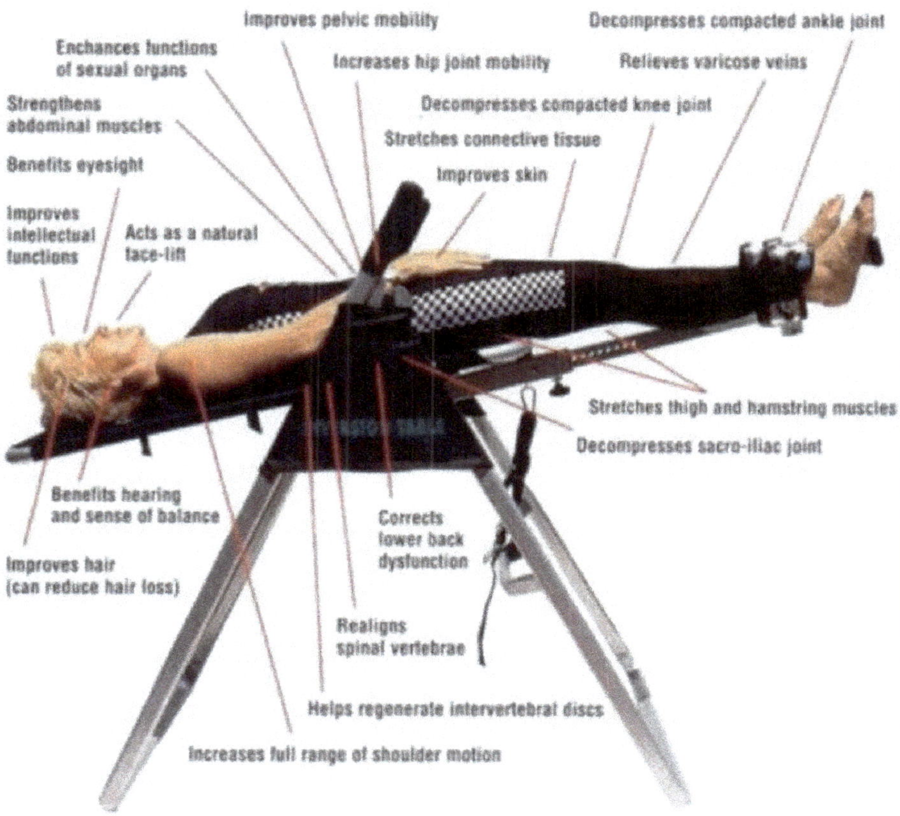

The picture to the left is an example of a perfect angle to start someone at. This gives them the benefits of the inversion table without some of the discomfort that comes from hanging full upside down...

As you may be already starting to tell, we are focusing a lot on the medical aspects of our work; however, the exercises you are learning about can be invaluable in your practice.

This exercise is a great example of what to do if a client comes in with an injury. We want you to start thinking outside of the box!

How can an inversion table be used as a great workout station?

How can you use this with your clients to train them for their sport of choice, aiding them in an increase in range of motion, strong core muscles, open and flexible joints, etc.?

WHAT KIND OF MEDICAL EXERCISE PROGRAM COULD YOU DEVELOP USING ONLY AN INVERSION TABLE?

In these images you see the bones of the skull and how the cervical spine fits into the skull at its axis.

How does exercising the muscles around the skull and upper cervical spine affect the rest of the spinal structure and your posture?

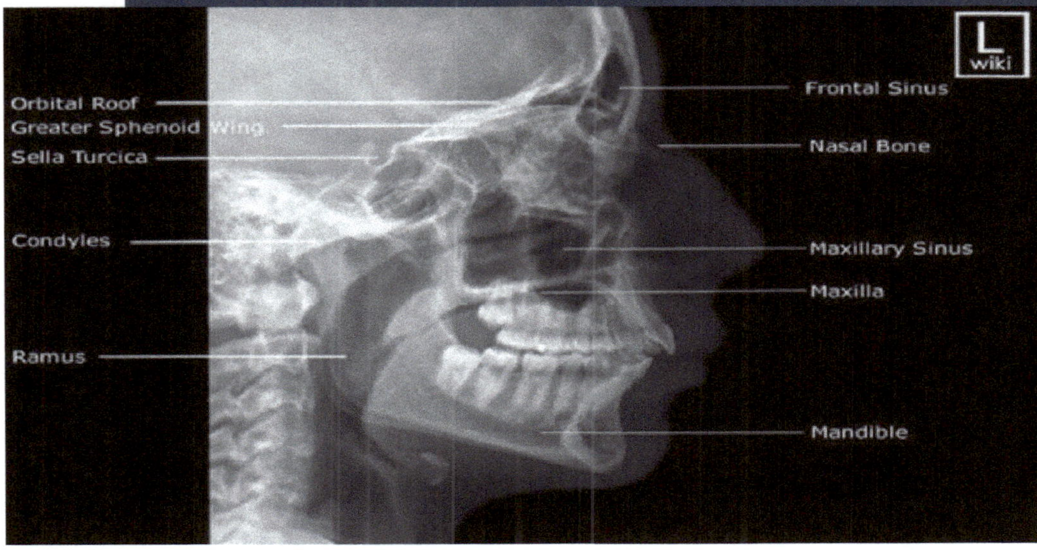

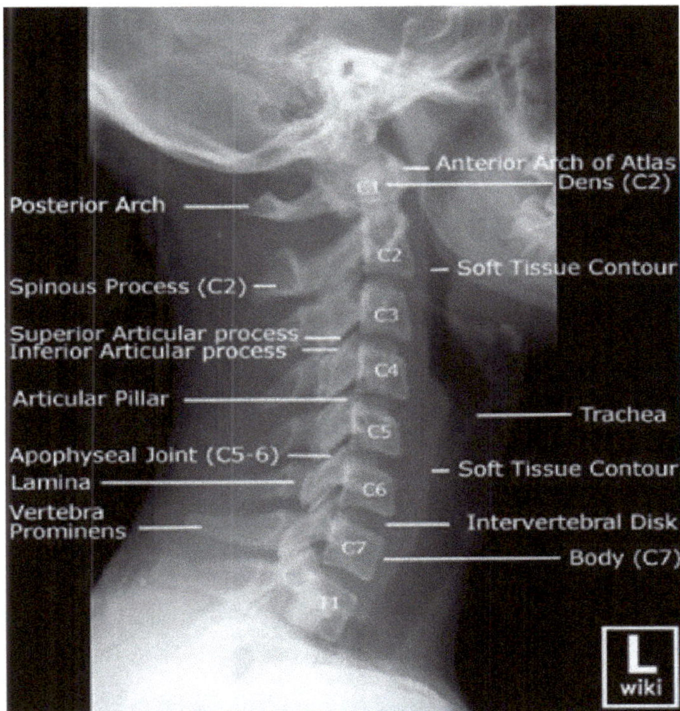

Although you are looking at an X-ray of a normal cervical spine, can you see which side of the neck is tighter rather than the other?

If you look at the very first image, you will see that there is a slight lean to the left. The outline of the musculature shows more space on the right than the left, and the right shoulder is higher than the left. These are subtle examples of what is possible to see when looking deeper at X-rays.

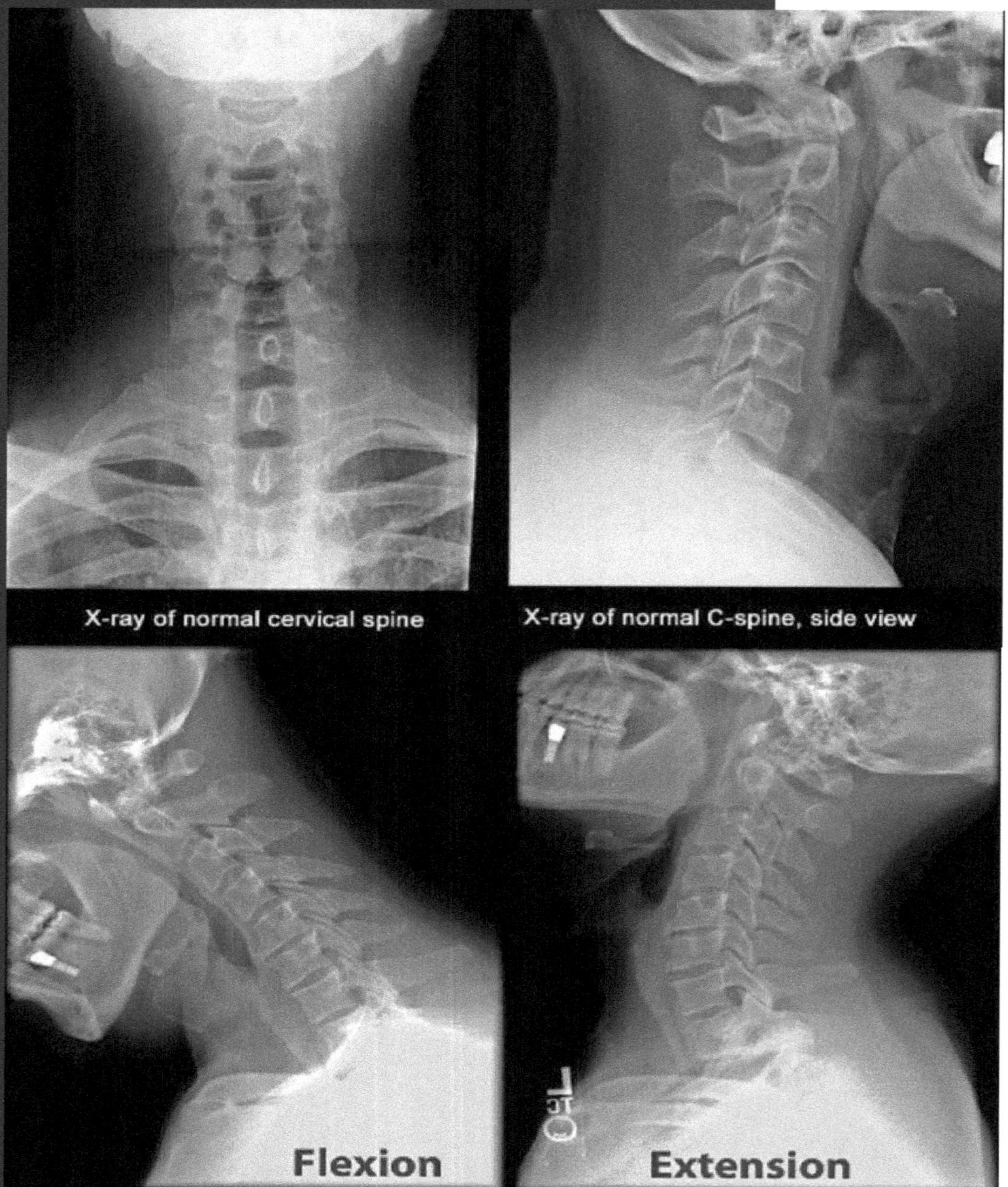

There are 12 muscles that make up the neck. These attach in places like your collar bone and into your shoulders. When they get tight, your entire upper body can stiffen. With MDRS you can increase range of motion and strength in the neck while helping to avoid future injury from occuring.

The rib cage houses our most precious organs. Lungs, heart, diaphragm, and liver are protected by our ribs. Each rib attaches to part of our spinal column. Creating exercises that increase strength and flexibility in the muscles that protect our rib cage is essential. The more flexibiity we have in our ribs, the more lung capacity we will have.

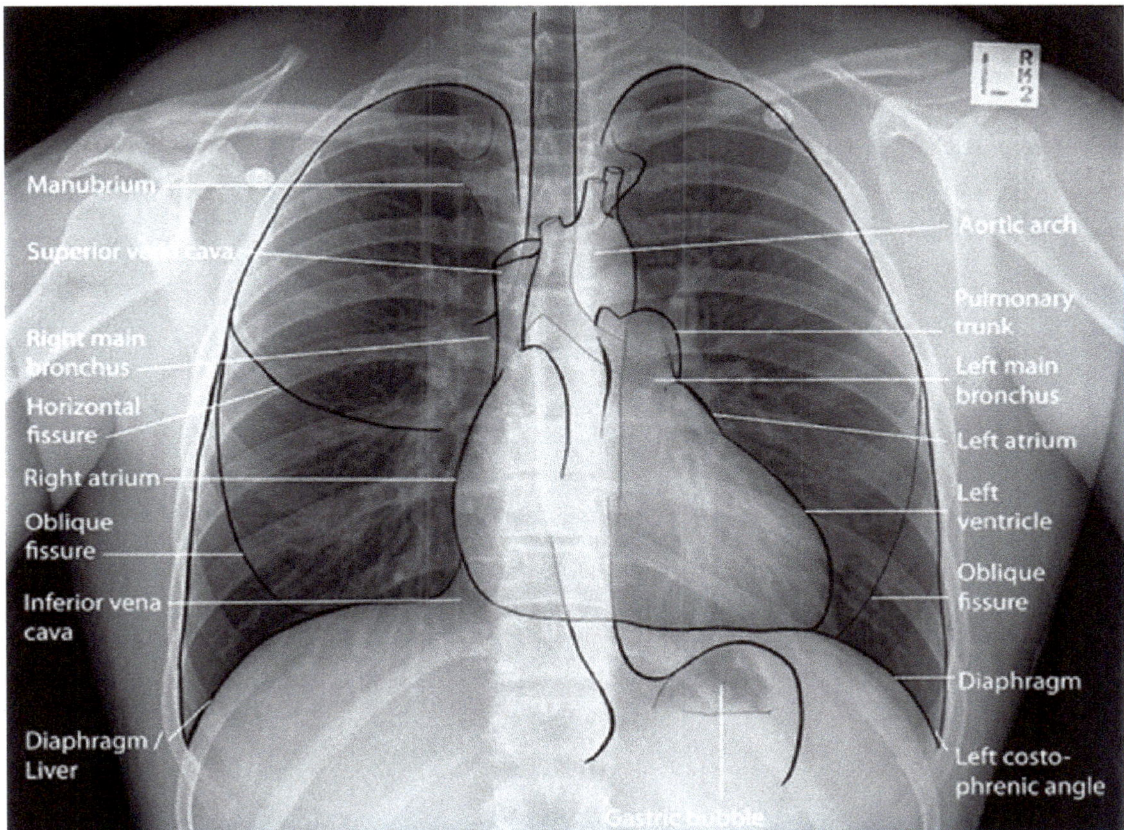

Not all X-rays are as clear as some that we have seen above. The following is a little more blurry which makes it more difficult to decipher. However there are some abnormalities that can be picked up.

Notice a slight degeneration of the disc between T10 and T11. You can see the narrowing of that space relative to the discs in the spaces below. The curvature going from L4 leading into L5, S1 joint is over-exaggerated which will cause this lower back arch to be greater. This can potentially be a cause for pain if posture is not great during workouts and even during everyday activities such as cooking or working at a desk.

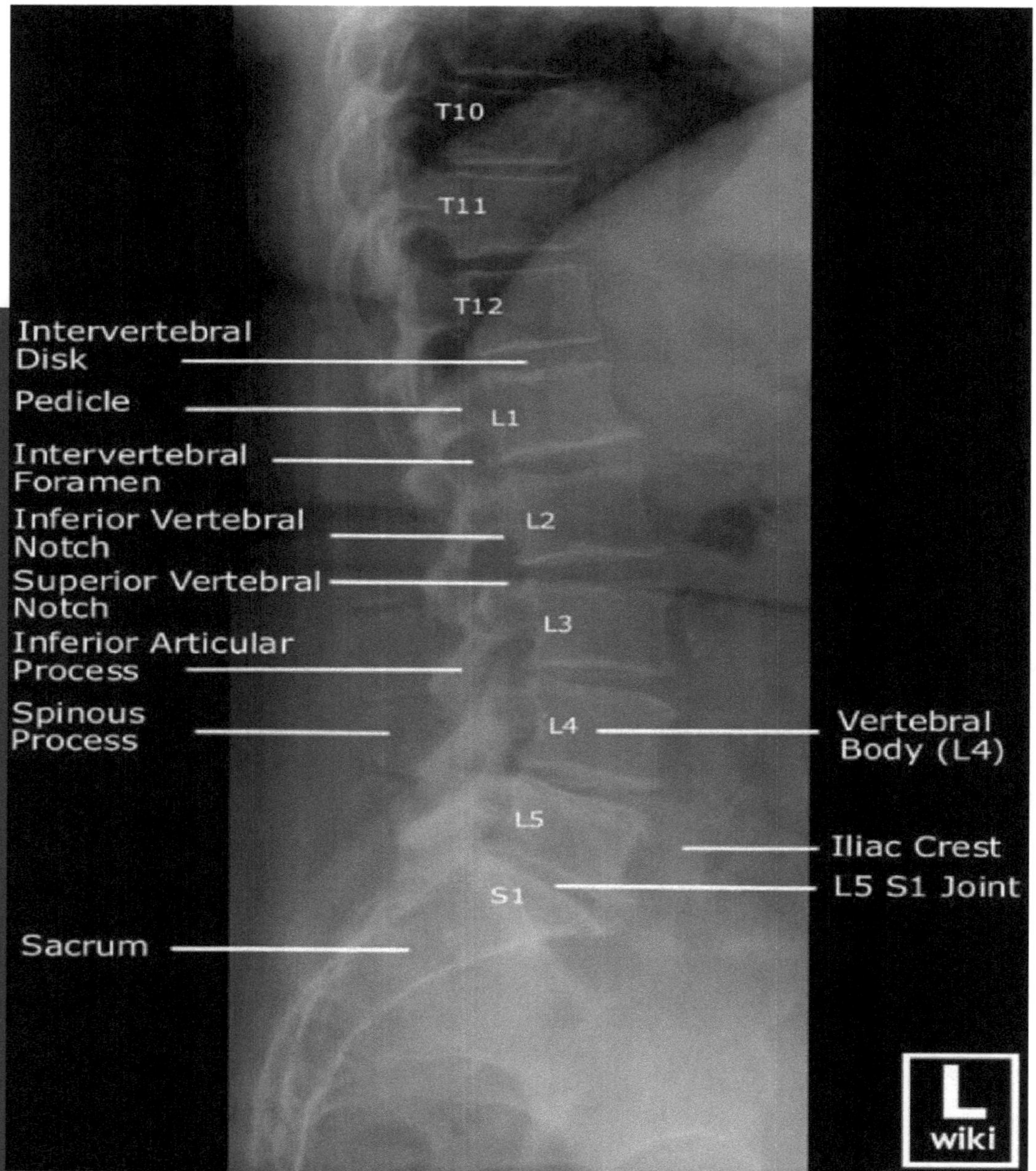

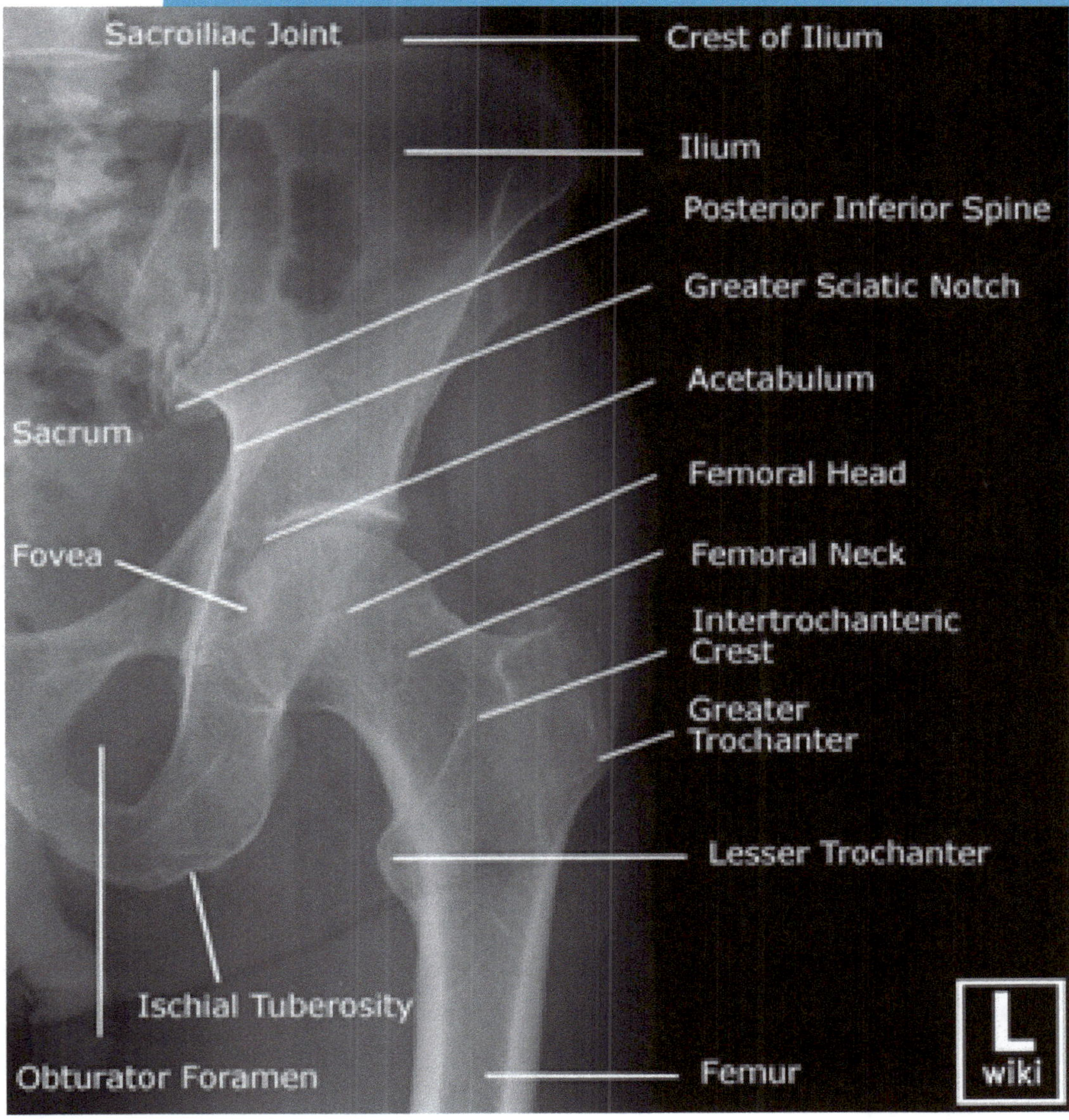

Hip replacement surgery is one of the most common problems that seniors deal with. They need highly-trained medical exercise professionals to strengthen them post surgery and, in many cases, help to prevent the need for surgery in the first place. Knowing how the muscles and attachments work will be essential to providing top quality care to this population.

Seventeen muscles make up the core of our body. They all attach in this bony structure. From groin pulls to strains and sprains to hips that make their way out of the socket, this is one of the most important parts of our kinesiology. How we move and our posture are both dependent on the amount of flexibility and power we have in our pelvic structure.

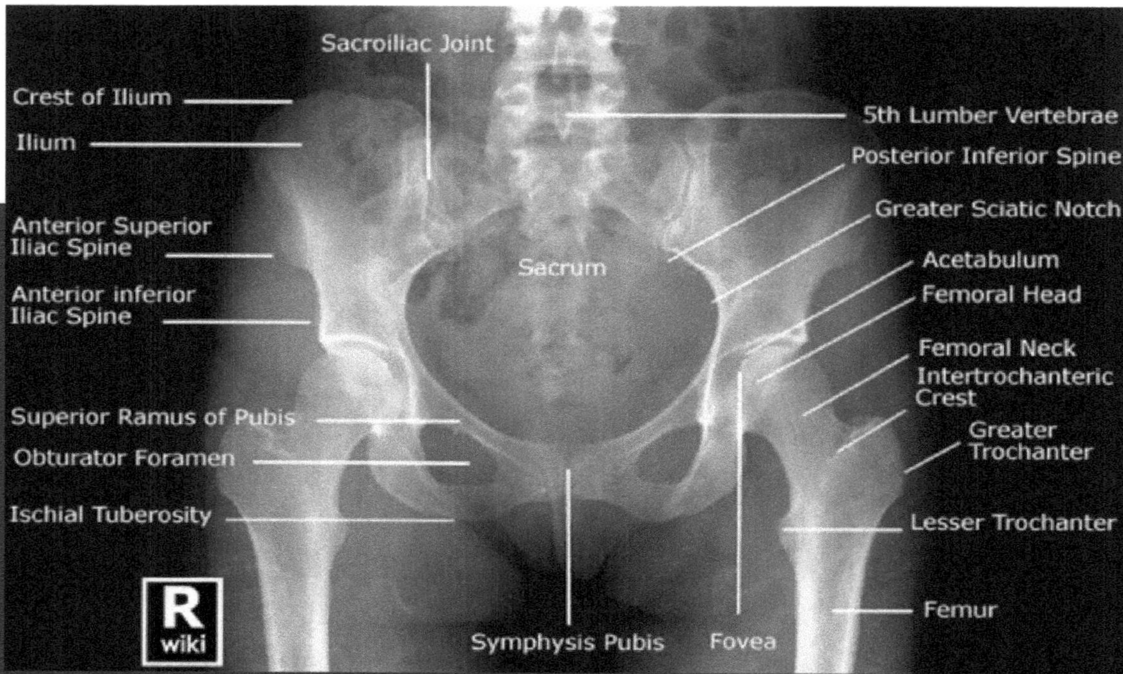
Sacroiliac Joint
Crest of Ilium
Ilium
Anterior Superior Iliac Spine
Anterior inferior Iliac Spine
Superior Ramus of Pubis
Obturator Foramen
Ischial Tuberosity
R wiki
Symphysis Pubis
Fovea
5th Lumber Vertebrae
Posterior Inferior Spine
Greater Sciatic Notch
Sacrum
Acetabulum
Femoral Head
Femoral Neck
Intertrochanteric Crest
Greater Trochanter
Lesser Trochanter
Femur

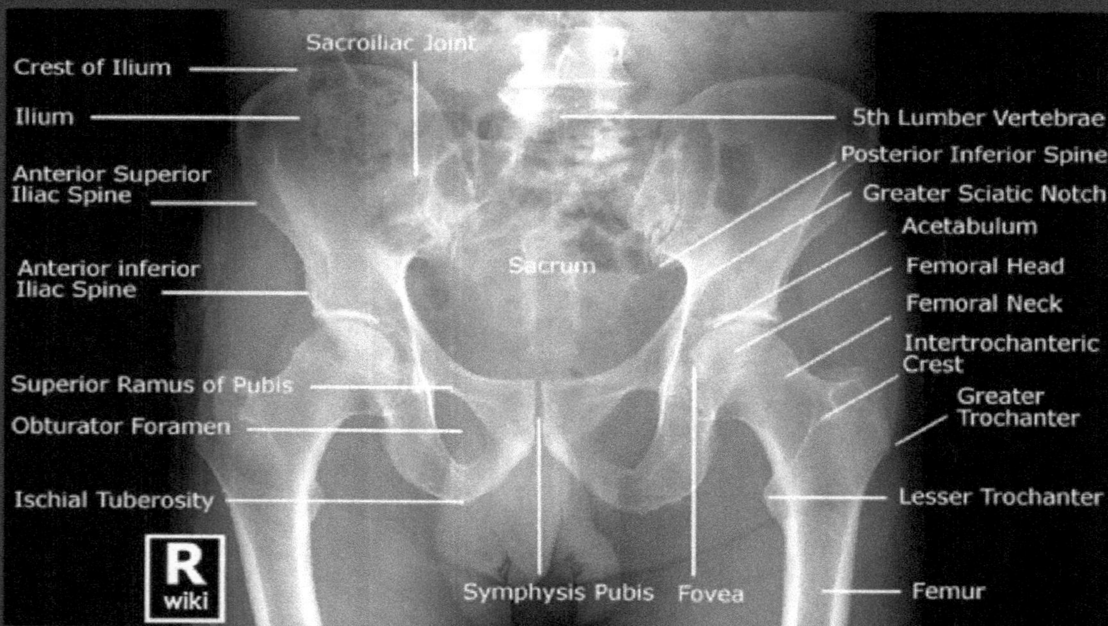
Sacroiliac Joint
Crest of Ilium
Ilium
Anterior Superior Iliac Spine
Anterior inferior Iliac Spine
Superior Ramus of Pubis
Obturator Foramen
Ischial Tuberosity
R wiki
Symphysis Pubis
Fovea
5th Lumber Vertebrae
Posterior Inferior Spine
Greater Sciatic Notch
Sacrum
Acetabulum
Femoral Head
Femoral Neck
Intertrochanteric Crest
Greater Trochanter
Lesser Trochanter
Femur

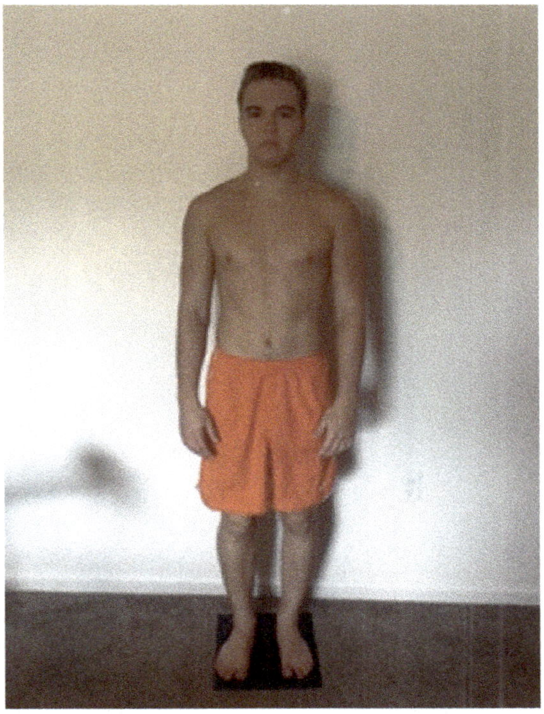

You can see that this side is fairly balanced with shoulders level and balanced hips all the way down to the toes.

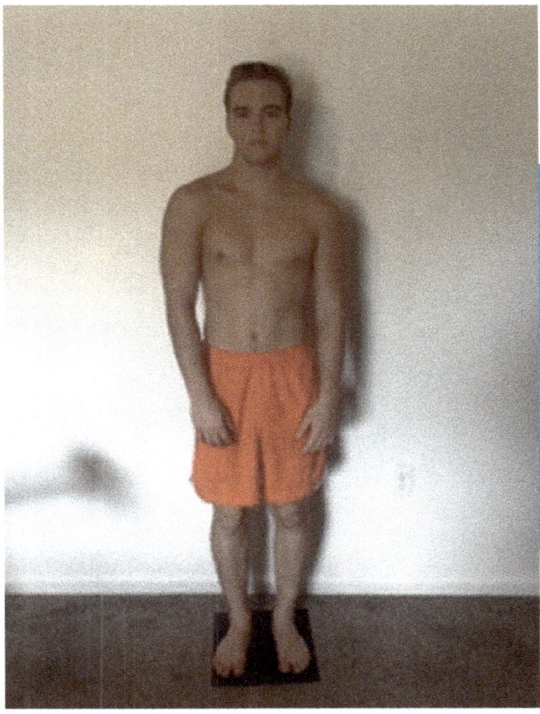

On this side the right shoulder is elevated and slightly turned in while the left side has a drop and turns back towards the wall.

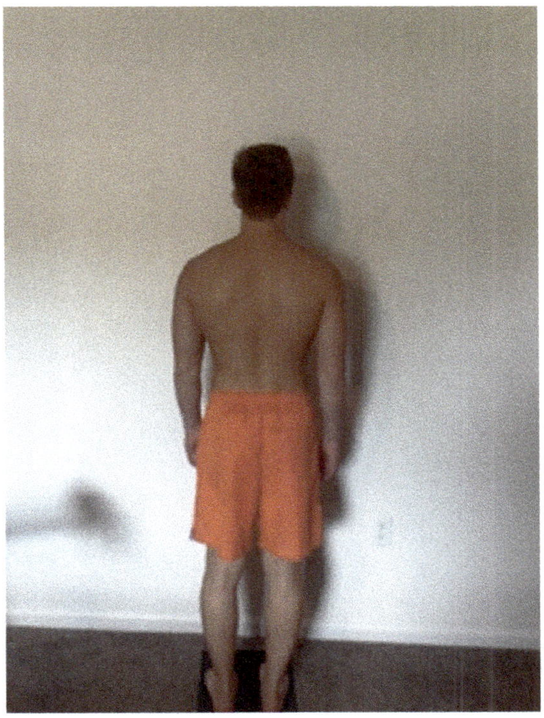

Again on this side there is a more balanced musculature. Slight imbalances in head position and angle; however the imbalances are insignificant.

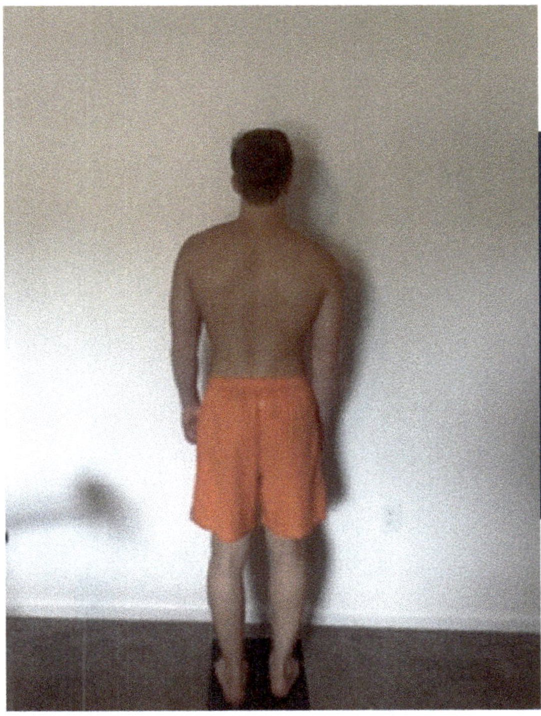

In this case the left shoulder is elevated and turned in. The shoulder blades are uneven and compensation in the lower frame is happening in the hips.

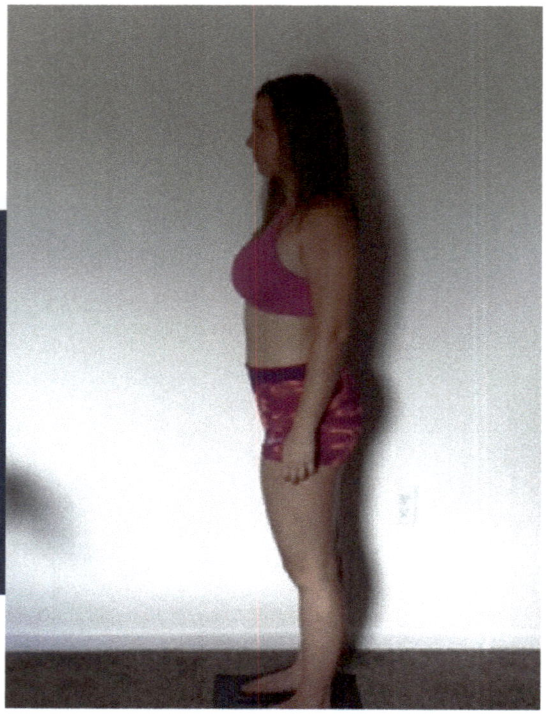

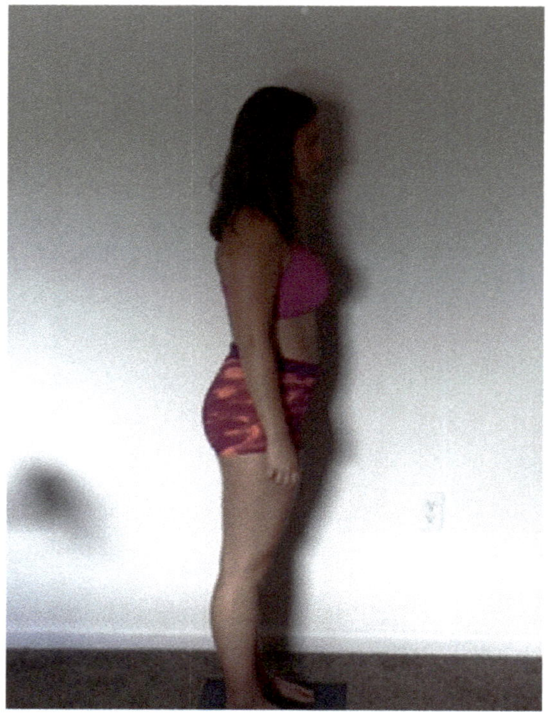

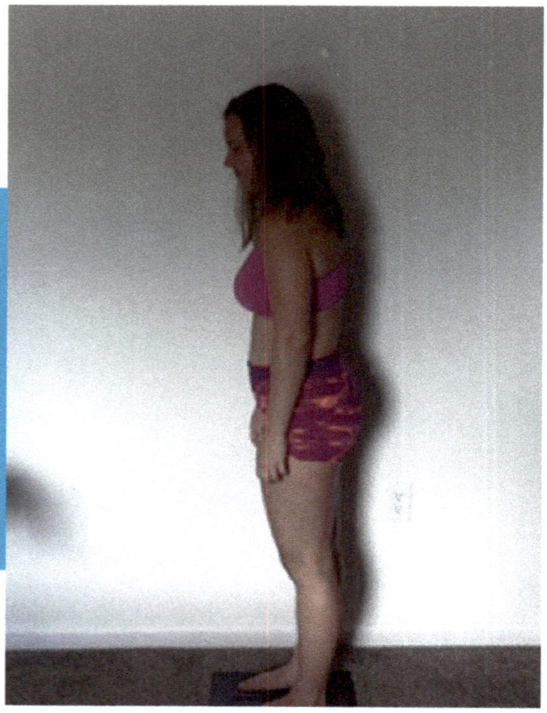

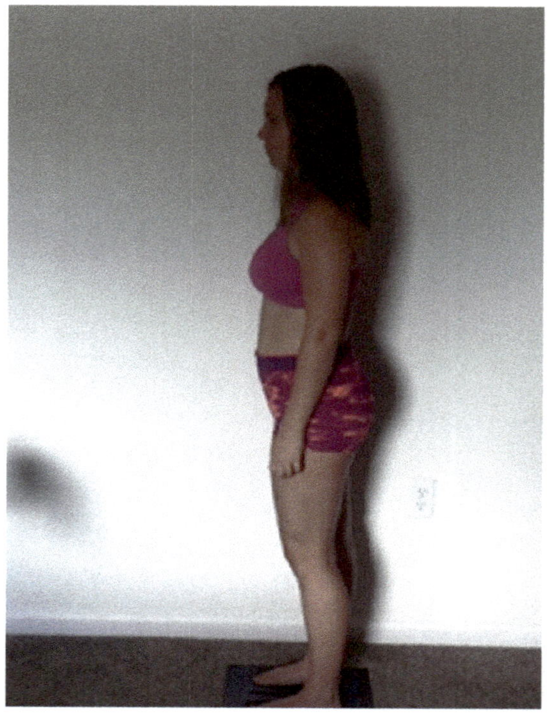

In the upper picture client is straight with arms back. Her left knee and foot is slightly turned out. Lower picture depicts upper thoracic and cervical issue.

In the upper picture the sway in her low back is distinct. What is difficult to see in these pictures, however, is that there are slight abnormalities in hip and pelvic alignment. See if you can spot them.

IN SUMMARY

During this module we dove into a new way of evaluation. We experienced a process in which each of us as practitioners can gain a deeper level of understanding about the human body as well as our own abilities to follow our intuition.

We learned a basic philosophy with regard to lab work and how to read the labs for a greater understanding of our clients' needs. We learned the difference between Pathological and Functional ranges and were able to experience the expertise of other modalities.

We learned the basics of reading of images - X-ray and MRI - and how to use that knowledge combined with our intuition in a way that both serves our clients at a higher level and also lets us be proactive with regards to injury prevention. If we know what the images tell us, we can train accordingly.

We used our 5 senses and the knowledge we gain with them and then added the sixth sense of intuition in order to create action steps that make the greatest gains.

DISCUSSION:

Describe at least three things you learned about yourself that you didn't already know.

Describe at least three things that you can take away from this experience that you can immediately implement in your practice.

How did it feel to completely lose the sense of sight?

List at least three specific ways your personal practice will benefit from this module.

By seeing the X-rays, you gained extra insights into the body at a deeper level than previously. What was the most profound thing you learned?

CHART TO SUCCESS IN EVALUATION

Skill Learned	How to Incorporate in Your Training	Notes

EVALUATION FORMS

All Level I **Evaluation Forms** are provided in Appendix A of this manual. You can print them and use them in your business.

Forms are available exclusively to workshop attendees & access is provided in your email box to Performance Therapy Academy back office HUB

LEVEL I: MODULE II

INTRODUCTION TO MULTI-DIRECTIONAL RESISTANCE STRETCHING© - LOWER BODY

MODULE II:
INTRODUCTION TO MULTI-DIRECTIONAL RESISTANCE STRETCHING© - LOWER BODY

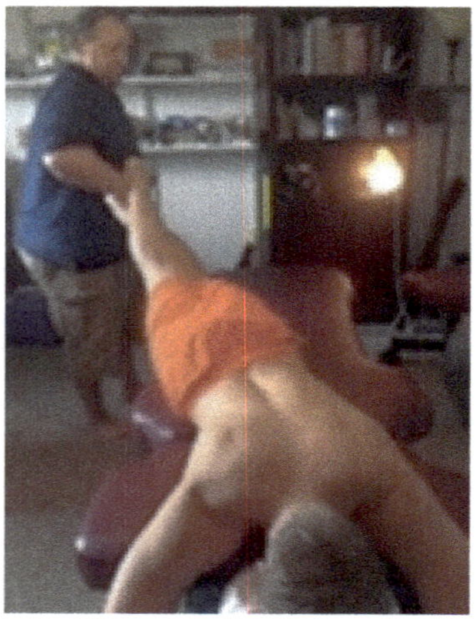

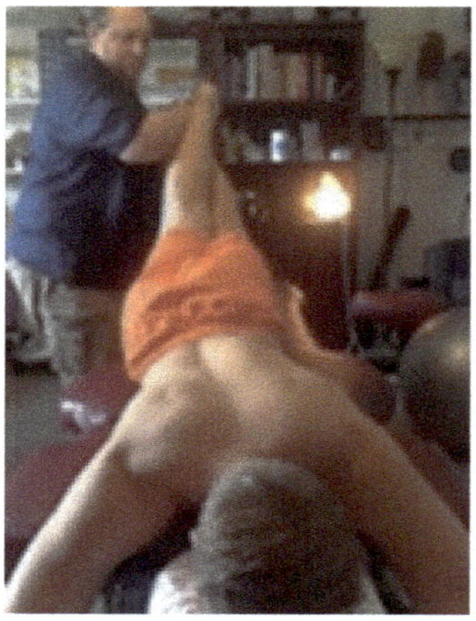

While stretching means different things to different people, for the purpose of this module we will define stretching as

"To stretch oneself by extending the limbs and lengthening the muscles to the utmost."

There are many forms of stretching that can be utilized together. Some techniques have been found to be much more effective than others.

KINDS OF STRETCHING

PASSIVE STRETCHING	an external force exerted upon the limb to move it into the new position
ACTIVE STRETCHING	eliminates force and its adverse effects from stretching procedures
STATIC STRETCHING	used to stretch muscles while the body is at rest
DYNAMIC STRETCHING	utilizing momentum from form, static-active stretching strength, and the momentum from static-active stretching strength
BALLISTIC STRETCHING	INEFFECTIVE AND PROBLEMATIC - CAUSING INJURIES
RESISTANCE STRETCHING	form of stretching in which a muscle simultaneously contracts and elongates

Our definition of the way MOST people normally stretch looks like this:

A single directional movement that takes a joint or muscle to the extreme of its range of motion, opening the muscle fibers, and creating space in your body.

NORMAL STRETCHING

This kind of stretching is most common among the few who actually take time out to stretch. It is a basic set of techniques that open up space allowing for a greater range of motion and less likely chance for injury.

POOR STRETCHING

We have all seen people out on a field or in a class doing the "Ballistic Stretching" The best literal illustration we can give for this is someone standing straight and trying to touch their toes, bouncing up and down. This uses bouncing motion to stretch muscles past their range of motion before they are ready to do so. This is not only poor stretching, but it can cause injury and should not be utilized.

NO STRETCHING

As seen in the couch potato.

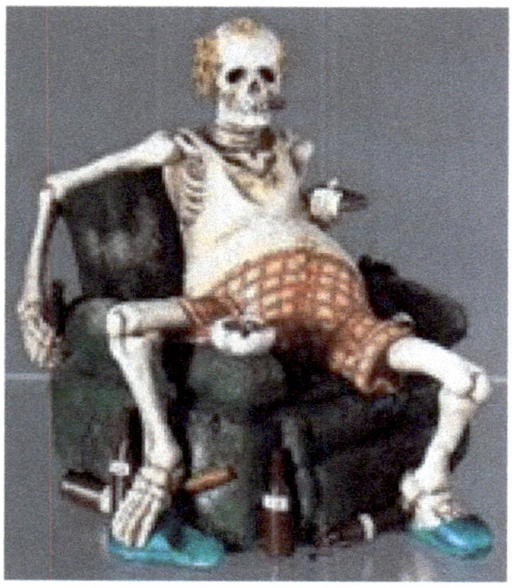

Coaching and playing with an adult baseball league, we would watch how maybe 90% of the players that come out to the field don't stretch, they simply start throwing and warming up. This lack of proper stretching is prevalent in most of our culture. It is a direct cause of almost all strain/sprain injuries as well as tears and dislocations.

Turning traditional exercises into

Multi Directional Resistance Stretching

came after years of working to combine the benefits of massage, physical therapy, personal training, and martial arts into an ultimately effective way to bring elite athletes out of the pain and sometimes despair of injury, and get them back into the game at a level they hadn't known before. We have always said that after an injury you not only can get back to where you were, you can always exceed your expectations with proper training and mindset.

Do you believe that someone can come out of injury better than ever?

Traditionally when an athlete became injured, he/she would go to a surgeon, a physical therapist, a massage therapist, and an athletic trainer or personal trainer. This was in addition to the normal coach and sport-specific trainer they would be seeing. This is quite a lot of different people that take up time, effort, and energy that otherwise could be spent in training.

> *"Out of a desire to be everything for everyone, minus the surgeon, I studied the body and how it reacted to palpation, movement, force or resistance, passive therapy, active therapy, kinesiology - both applied and educational, as well as electronic therapies such as electric stimulation via pulse machines, and even cold laser treatment. I wanted to know what would create the fastest, most exponential healing process while at the same time developing more strength, power, and flexibility so that the athletes I worked with could not only return to playing, they could deliver a performance far exceeding what even they thought was possible."*
>
> **Ari Gronich, The Performance Therapist**

Traditional use of a therapy table was the perfect place to begin working, and it is where we begin today.
(If we don't have enough tables, we can work on the floor using exercise or yoga mats).

INTERACTIVE ASSESSMENT DRILL

Equipment needed for this section will be weighted power balls (3, 5, 7, 10, 12 lb. and up depending on client), a 55cm – 75cm exercise ball, and a 3 lb. yoga ball.

The tools used will create a resistance that will intensify the stretching while recruiting balancer muscles and core muscles thereby working a larger area of muscle tissue at the same time as isolating a specific muscle, tendon, ligament, and/or joint group.

This is where looks and function separate. If you watch someone doing these movements, it looks simple; however, nothing can be farther from the truth. As Dominique Arnold, Olympic track star and American record holder once said,

"It gives me like Bruce Lee type strength and flexibility!!!"

We begin by assessing lower body abnormalities as well as taking a client through a series of exercises that will increase strength, flexibility, and power.

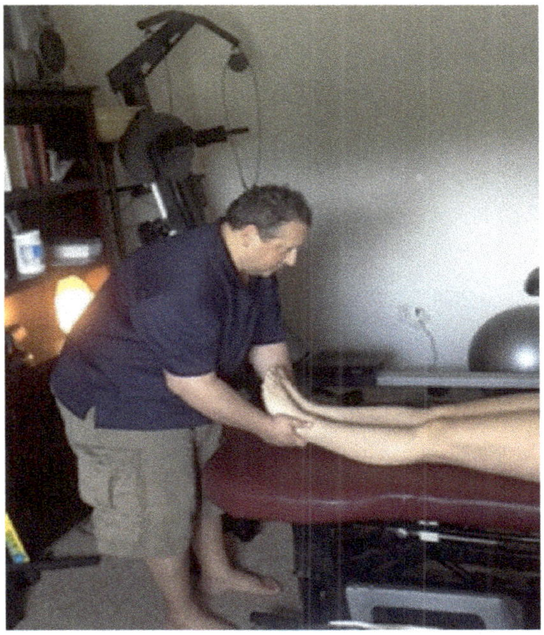

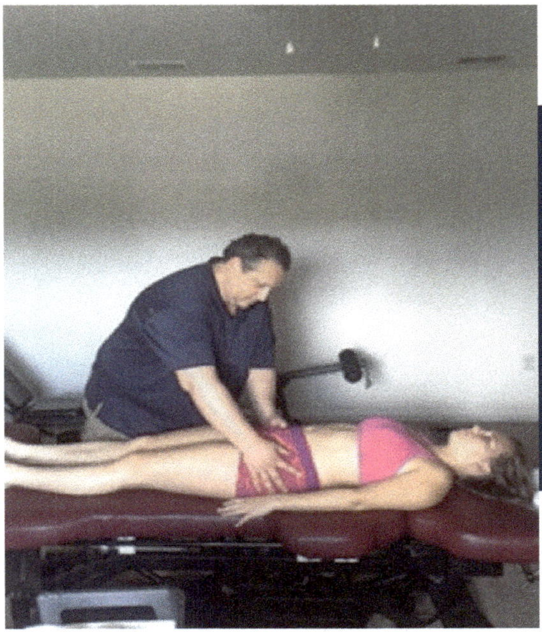

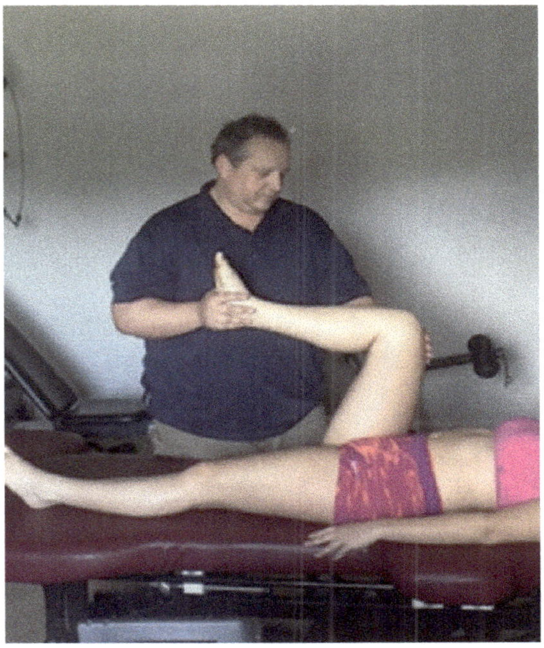

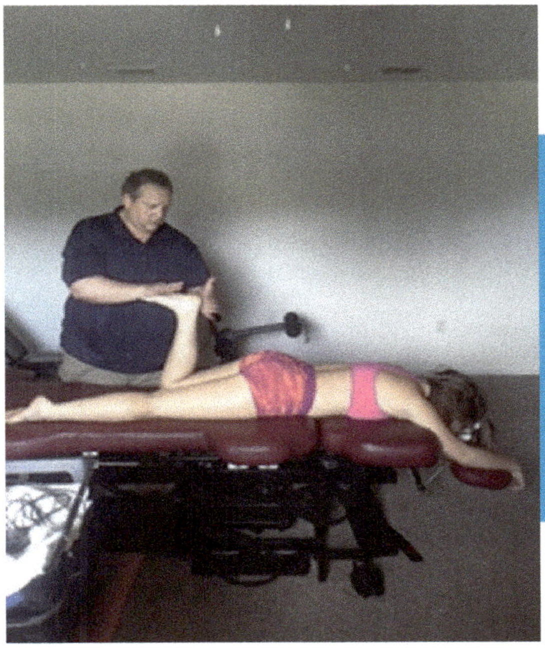

In the top picture we are assessing hip alignment. Check feet, ankles, and knees in order. Bottom picture, when lifting into position, does the knee want to go in, go out, or stay in alignment?

Upper Picture checking pelvic bones for alignment. Are they even in elevation, rotation, and muscular tension? Bottom picture shows tightness in Achilles as well as weakness in ad- or abductors depending on direction the foot wants to fall.

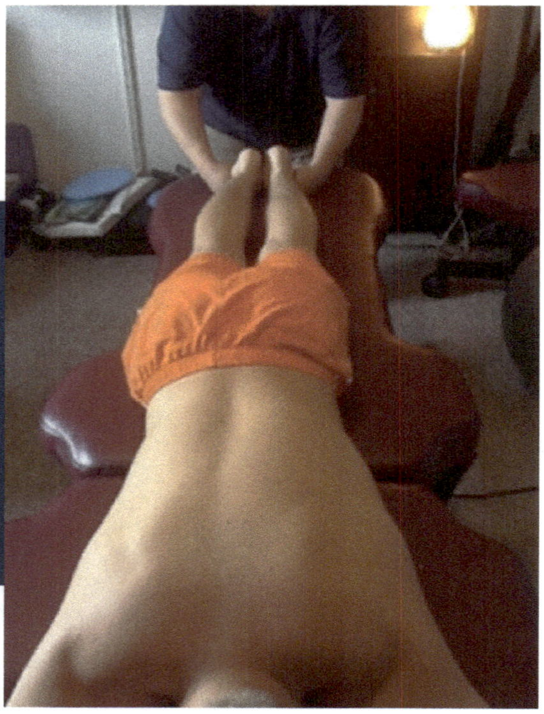

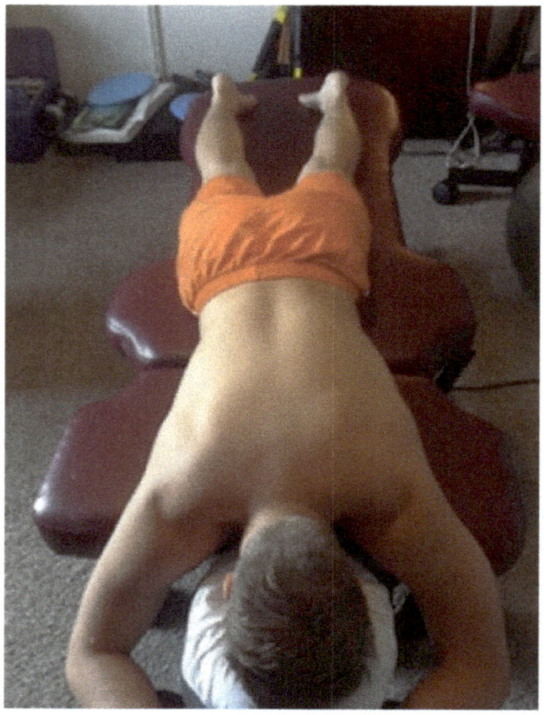

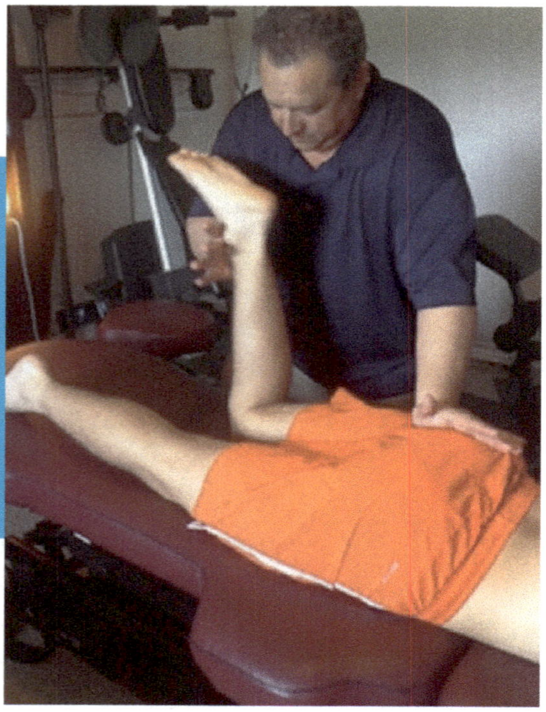

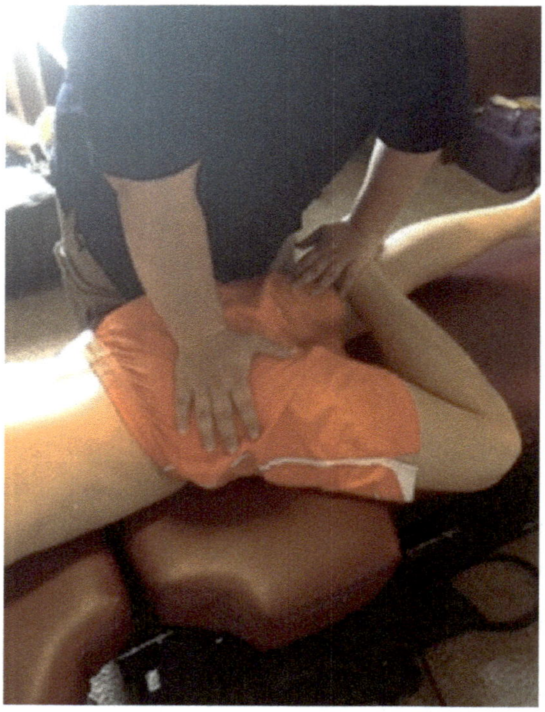

In the upper picture we are assessing hip to foot alignment. Check heels, behind knee, and pelvic bones for even alignment. In the bottom picture we bring the foot up to 90° to see if hips shift position or if the foot wants to go in or out, showing weakness.

Upper picture is a general head to toe assessment. Can you see that the left hip is slightly rotated? In the bottom picture we are assessing whether the hip joint has flexibility for internal rotation and at what point the pelvis will begin elevating.

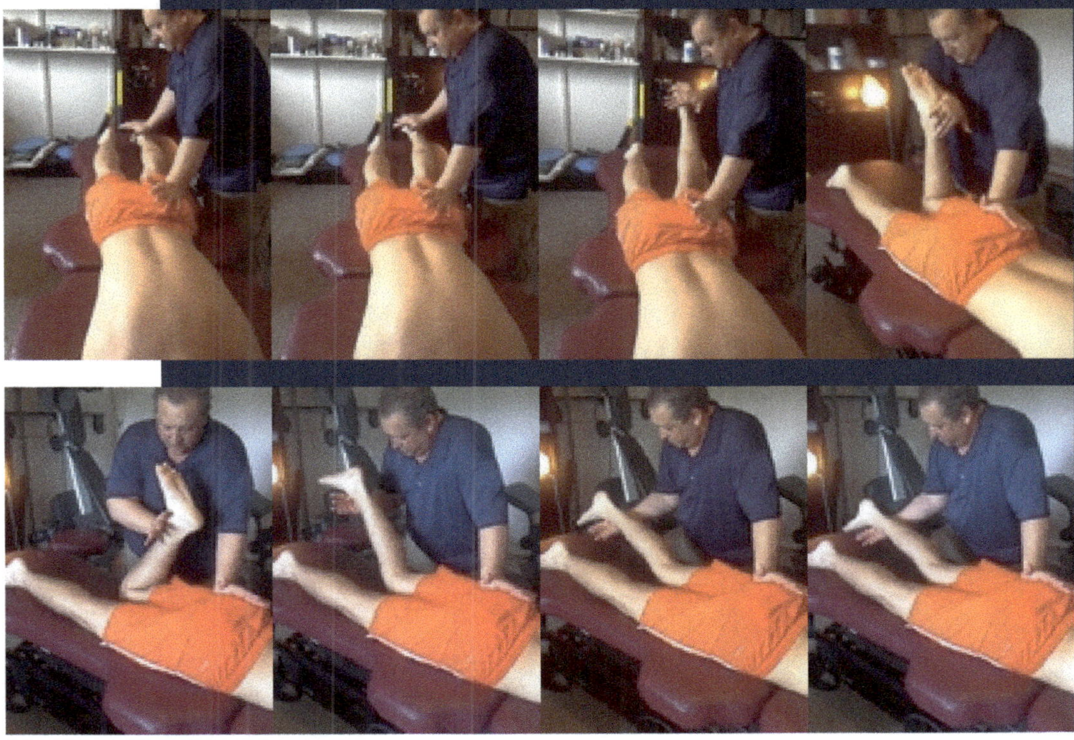

Stabilize hip with one hand while having client lift against resistance from the other hand. Only allow slow movement through the ROM in order to engage the most muscle fibers possible. This also allows for a much more thorough stretch of the opposing muscles. When the foot gets to its stopping point, encourage the client to push farther and hard squeezing the contraction while you resist. This will give the quad muscles as well as psoas a deeper stretch. Then reverse tension and have them push against your resistance all the way back down to the table. Make sure they fulfill this exercise in a continuous effort and do not give up - thus ensuring a more thorough engagement of all muscles' fibers.

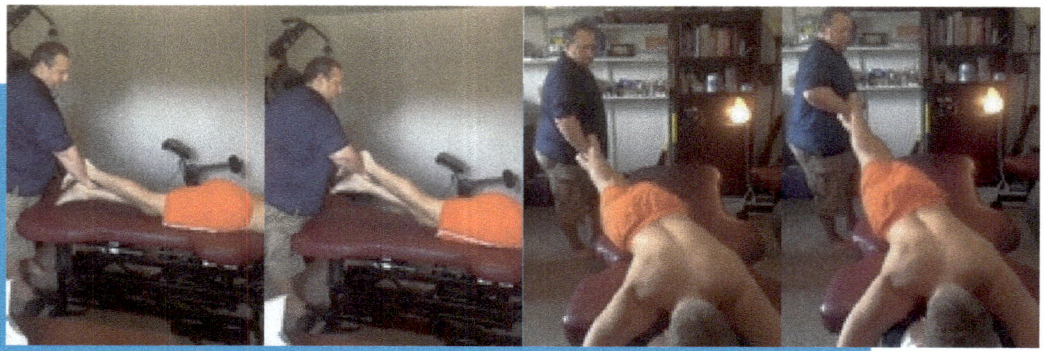

Cross feet and place your wrist or arm, whichever is more comfortable, in between and have client squeeze. While they squeeze, you are lifting their legs up off the table and then twisting them from side to side. This will engage ad- and abductors, groin, piriformis, glutes, and psoas as well as tibialis and calf muscles. When finished with one long repetition, have client switch which foot is on top and do it again.

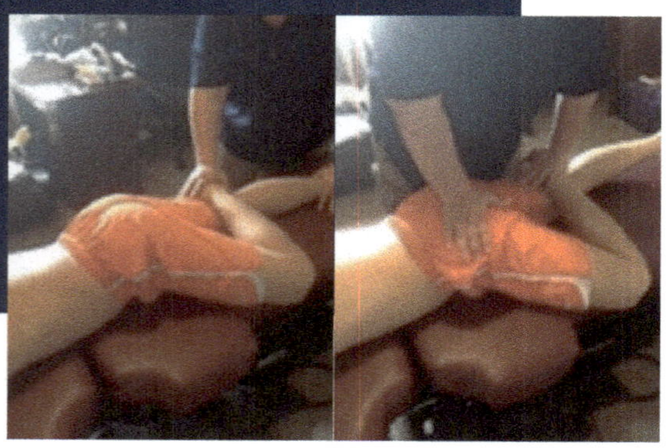

Place the ankle and instep of foot over the crease behind knee. Stabilize the hip with your other hand and create a deep stretch throughout glutes and psoas.

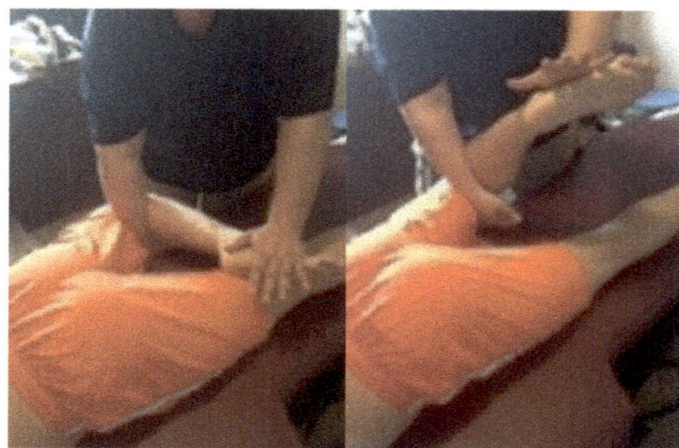

Place the heel of your hand in the crease behind the knee push down on the ankle of the foot and have the client rotate leg up. To enhance the effectiveness, place hand on ligament behind knee causing a deeper stretch.

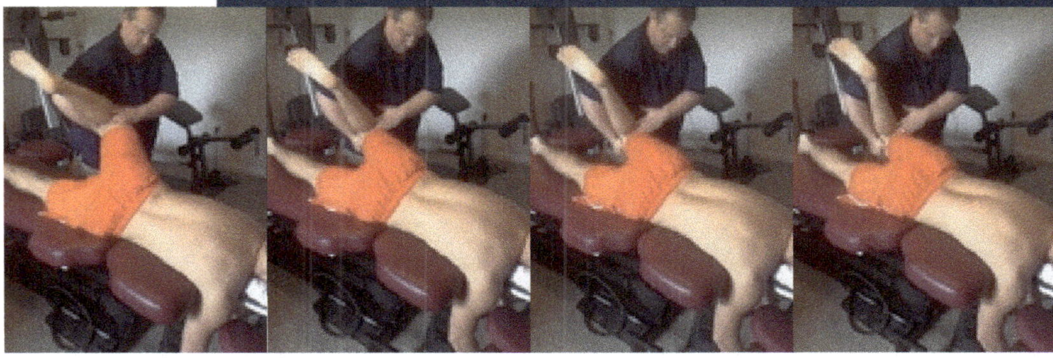

This groin/psoas stretch challenges the rotational aspects of the client's muscles as well as inner core strength. First grab at the knee and rotate leg to the outside of the body. Have the client rotate hips downward while giving steady resistance throughout ROM.

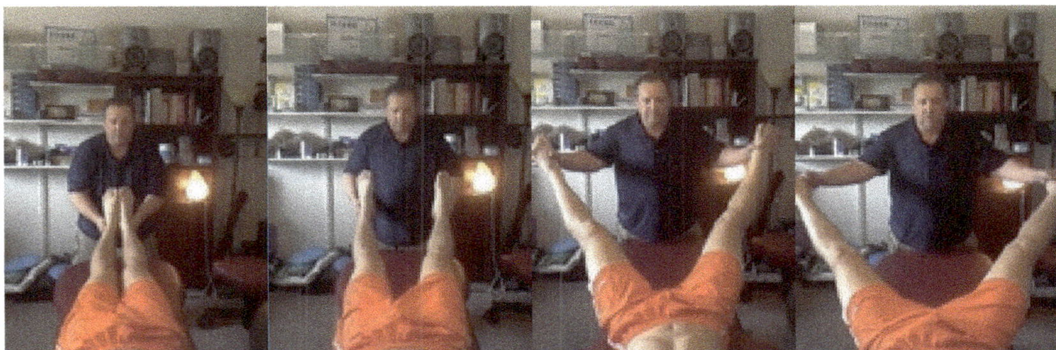

Hold feet together slightly off the table and simply resist as you have the client spreading legs. As they are spreading out, lift the legs up to a higher level engaging more muscle fibers and challenging the stabilizers. Once they get to the extent of their own ROM, push legs farther apart and have them squeeze against your resistance. As they are squeezing, you are beginning to lower the legs back down toward the table.

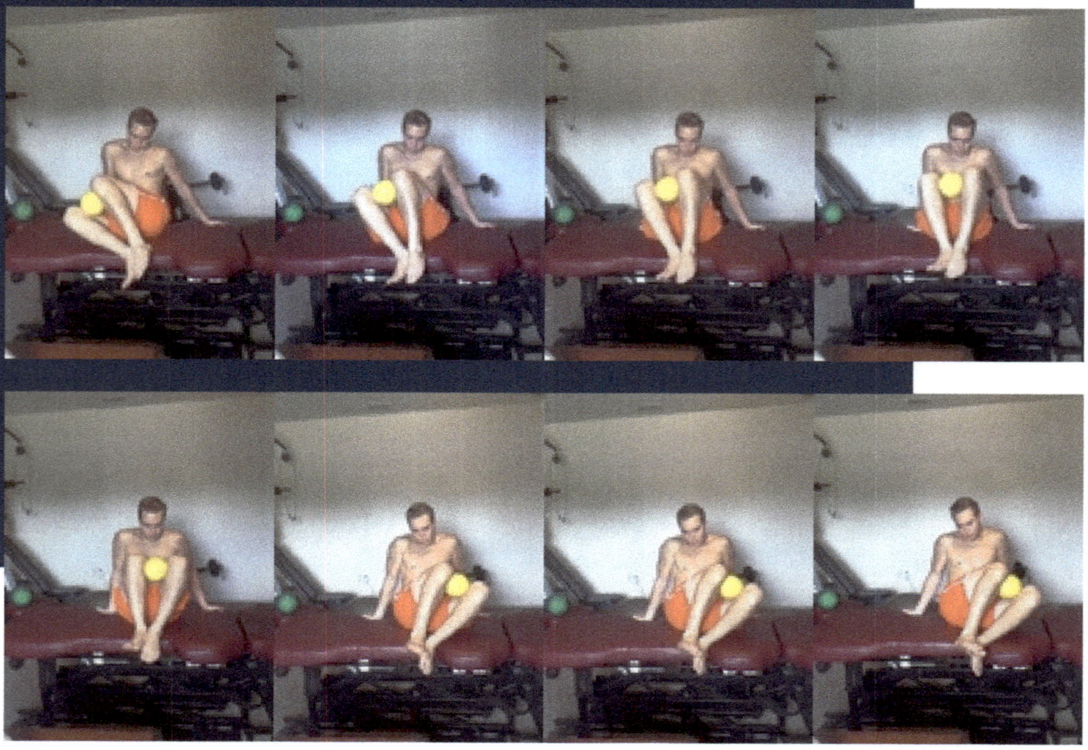

While sitting on the edge of the table balancing back on client's hands, put a weighted medicine ball between the legs. Lift feet up and twist the legs from side to side while squeezing the ball. This exercise will stretch lower torso and oblique muscles while stretching and contracting upper legs. It will challenge balance which also increases the recruitment of stabilizer muscles and, depending on how slowly they go, how hard the squeeze, and how long they can hold, client's muscle cell endurance will be increased.

IN SUMMARY

"You never have to get someone off of a table to give them an extremely thorough workout!"

Ari Gronich, The Performance Therapist

DISCUSSION:

What did you take away from this module that was the most powerful?

____

____

____

What did you learn that you can implement in your practice immediately?

____

____

____

What did you think could be altered or tweaked to make better?

____

____

____

LEVEL I: MODULE III

INTRODUCTION TO MULTI-DIRECTIONAL RESISTANCE STRETCHING© - UPPER BODY

MODULE III:
INTRODUCTION TO MULTI-DIRECTIONAL RESISTANCE STRETCHING© - UPPER BODY

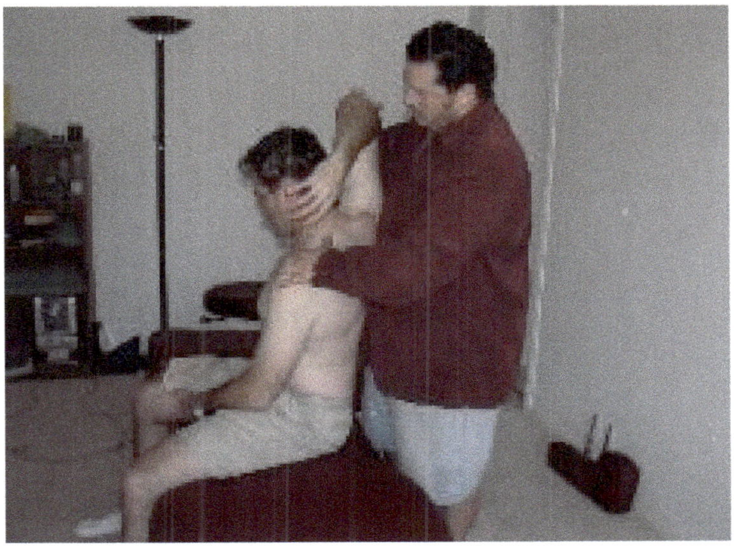

Stretching the upper body is slightly more delicate than stretching the lower body. Typical stretching as well as weight lifting happens in the linear aspects of the musculature rather than in the stabilizing muscles. This general way of training leaves several weak points in the system which are susceptible to injury. We must take this into account when working with clients.

How many of your clients cannot do exercises that you give them to do because of upper body injury?

How many clients a year do you lose to injury or pain?

As we went through the previous modules, we experienced the value of a great evaluation process. This expresses both what is happening in the body as well as guides what needs to happen for treatment and training protocols and will give you a great sense of where to go and what to do in order to stretch and strengthen these joints, ligaments, tendons, and muscles.

The balance that occurs with Multi-Directional Resistance© Stretching is significant. It helps to prepare the body for any eventuality by creating a balance between the strong and weak sides of the body so that one doesn't overpower the other.

Imagine you are left handed and typically stronger in that arm and hand; however, in this case you are holding your purse on your right side. Someone comes to grab that purse out of your hand and ends up pulling at your arm as you clench down on the purse. The training you are doing in this course would allow your normally weaker arm to be equally strong and flexible and, instead of having your arm ripped out of its socket, you are able to hold on to your purse and fight off the perpetrator with your other arm - saving your body from injury and your purse from theft.

If you are training an athlete, it does not matter which sport they are in. This work will increase their range of motion, power, muscle endurance, and speed while decreasing chances of injury and fatigue. This combination will inevitably lengthen the career of any athlete.

INTERACTIVE DRILL

We will begin this section going through the upper body testing for weakness and imbalances, then move into the exercise portion of this module.

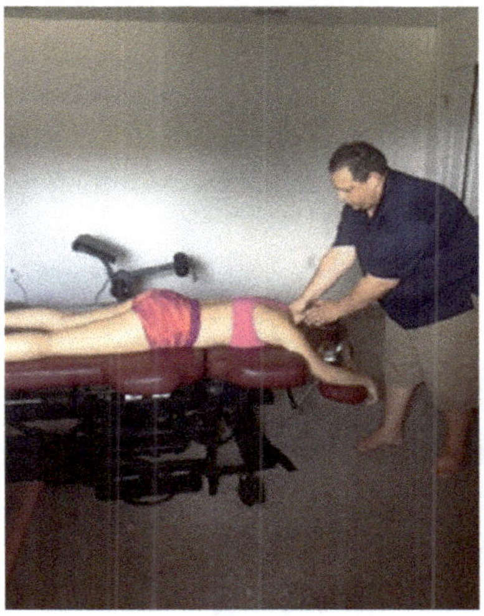

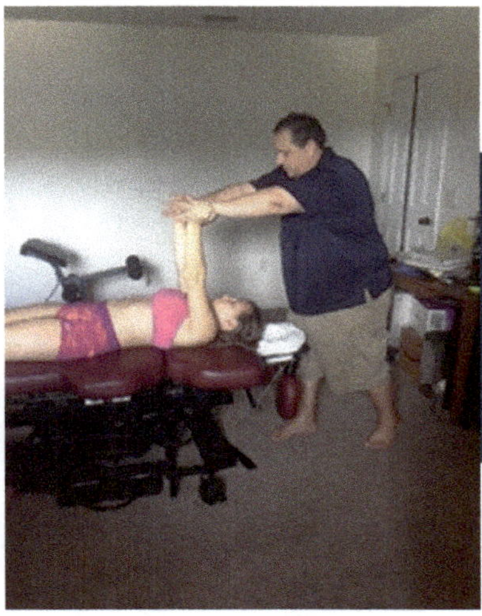

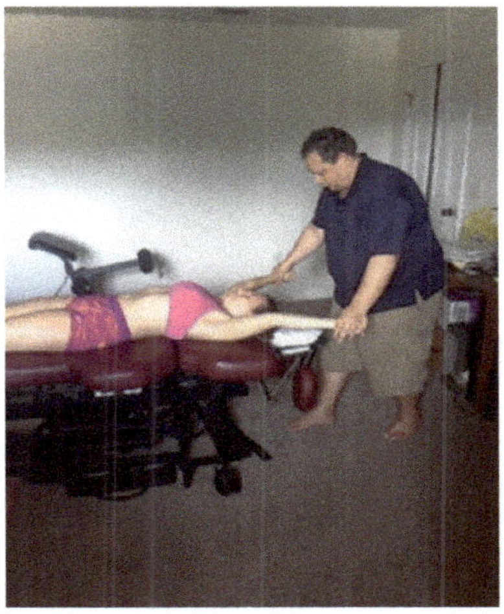

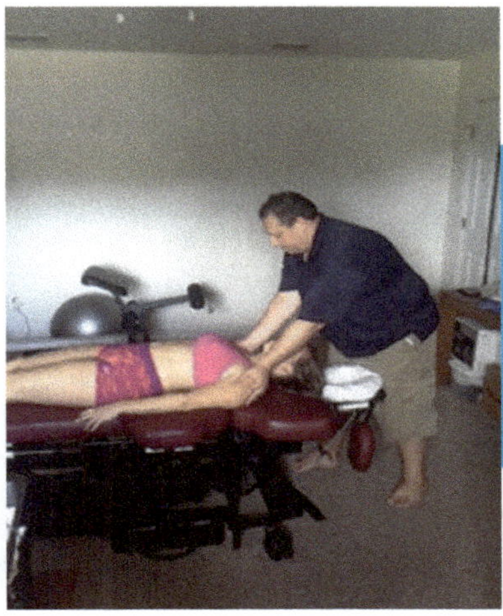

In the upper picture we are checking the cervical spine for alignment through to the hips. Bottom picture is checking rotation of shoulder blades through an elevated position and can demonstrate spinal muscle imbalances if low back begins to arch.

Upper picture we are testing strength and balance between both shoulders by isolating the movement. Patient is squeezing slightly against the resistance of therapist hands. Bottom picture is checking shoulder tension and position as well as cervical alignment.

THIS WILL BE A HANDS-ON PORTION AS WELL AS INTERACTING WITH THE PICTURES BELOW!!!

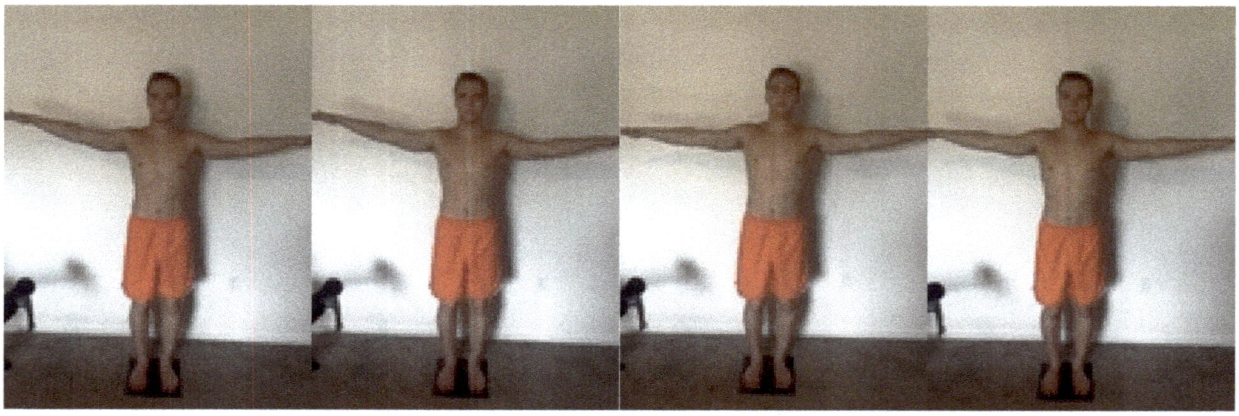

CAN YOU TELL WHERE THE IMBALANCE IS IN EACH OF THE PICTURES ABOVE?

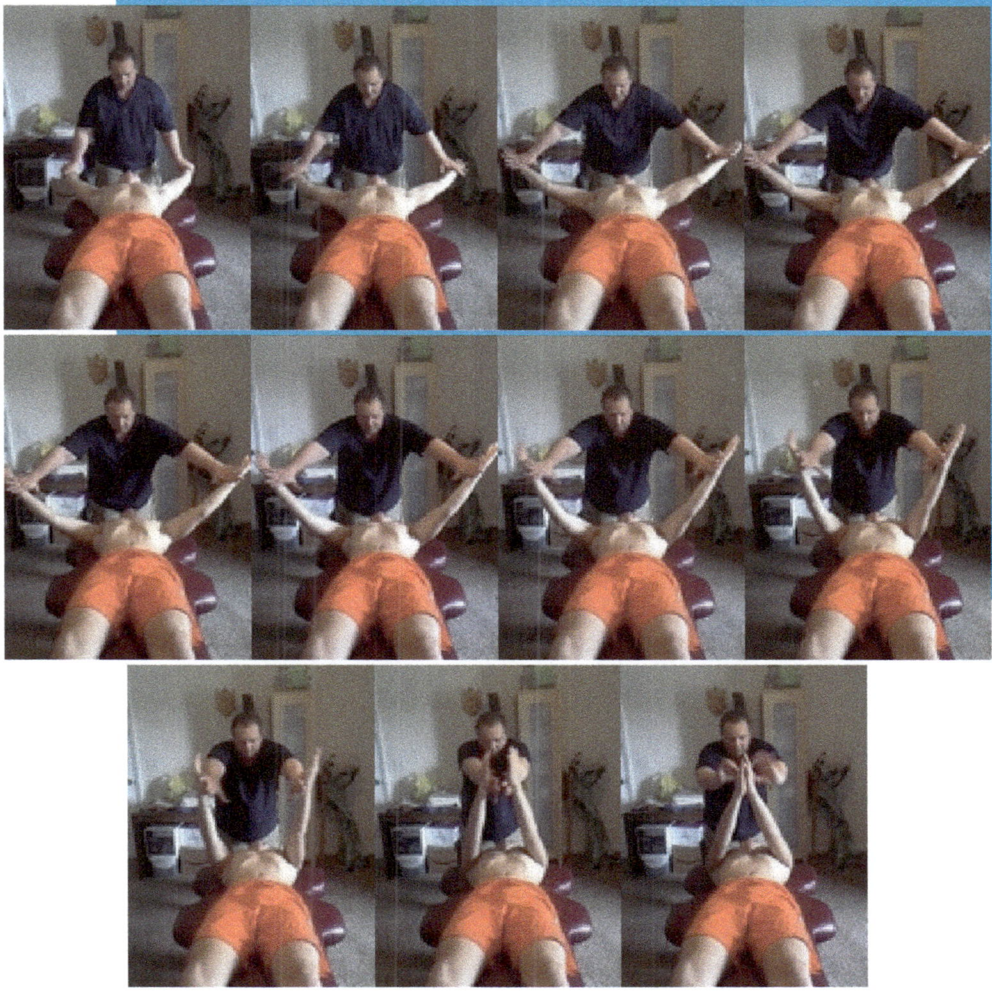

Exercises for shoulders, chest, and upper core. Trainer is resisting the movement as well as guiding client throughout the range of motion. Not only does this work out the client, but it allows you as a trainer to really sense where imbalances are in the range of motion which allows you to evaluate and diagnose possible injuries or damage.

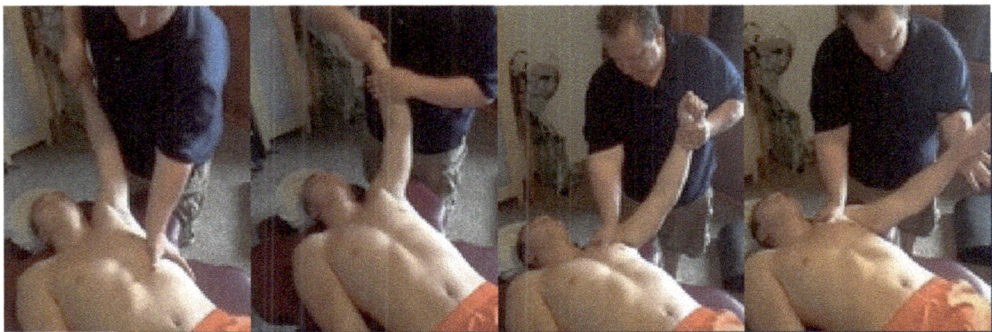

Exercise for single shoulder to isolate shoulders, chest, and upper core. By doing single side as well as both sides, you can eliminate compensation from one side or the other.

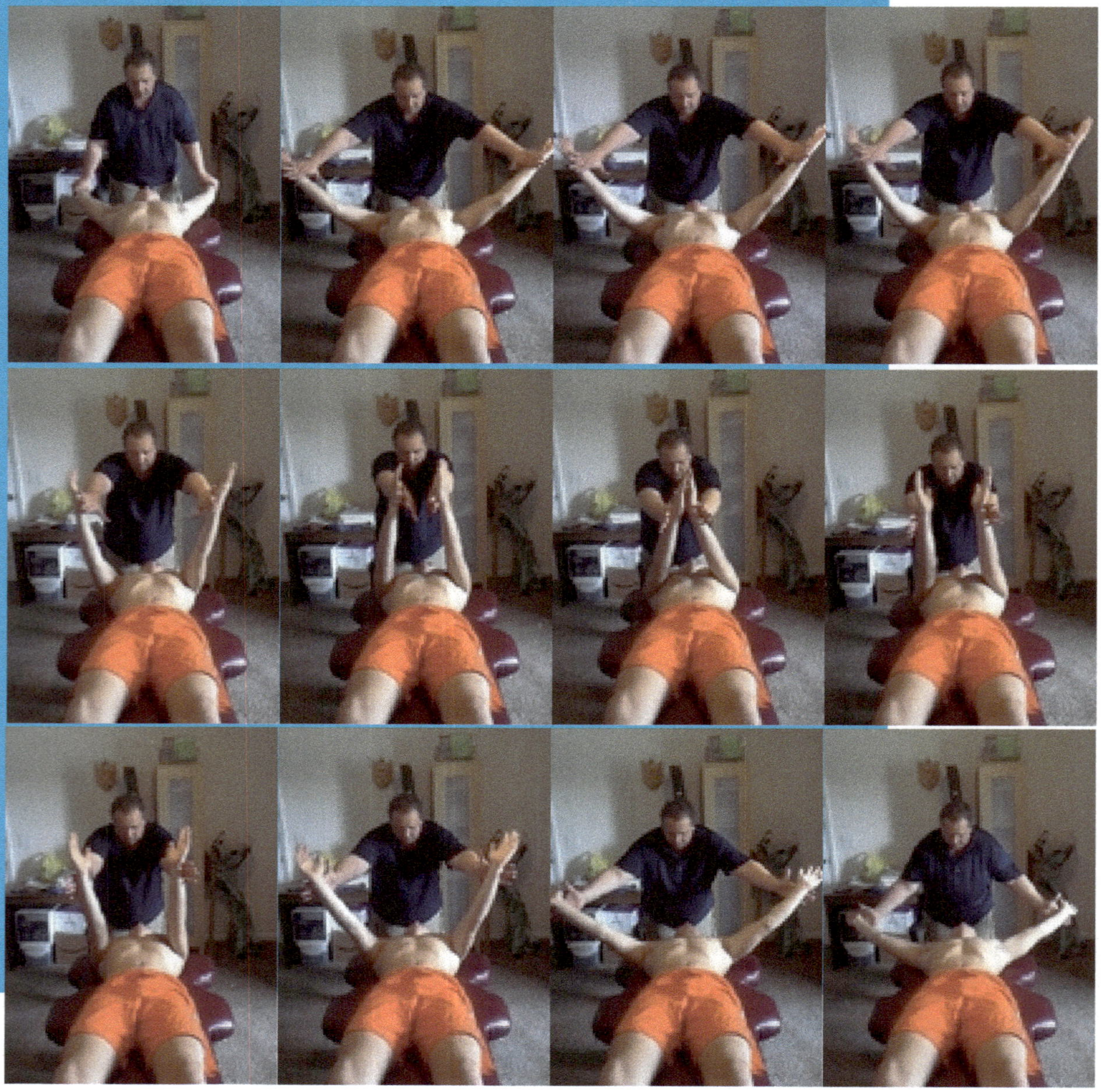

This is a full ROM circular exercise. Rather than straight up and down, we are going from straight back around the sides and up to centerline and back. This works the entire ROM of the rotator cuffs.

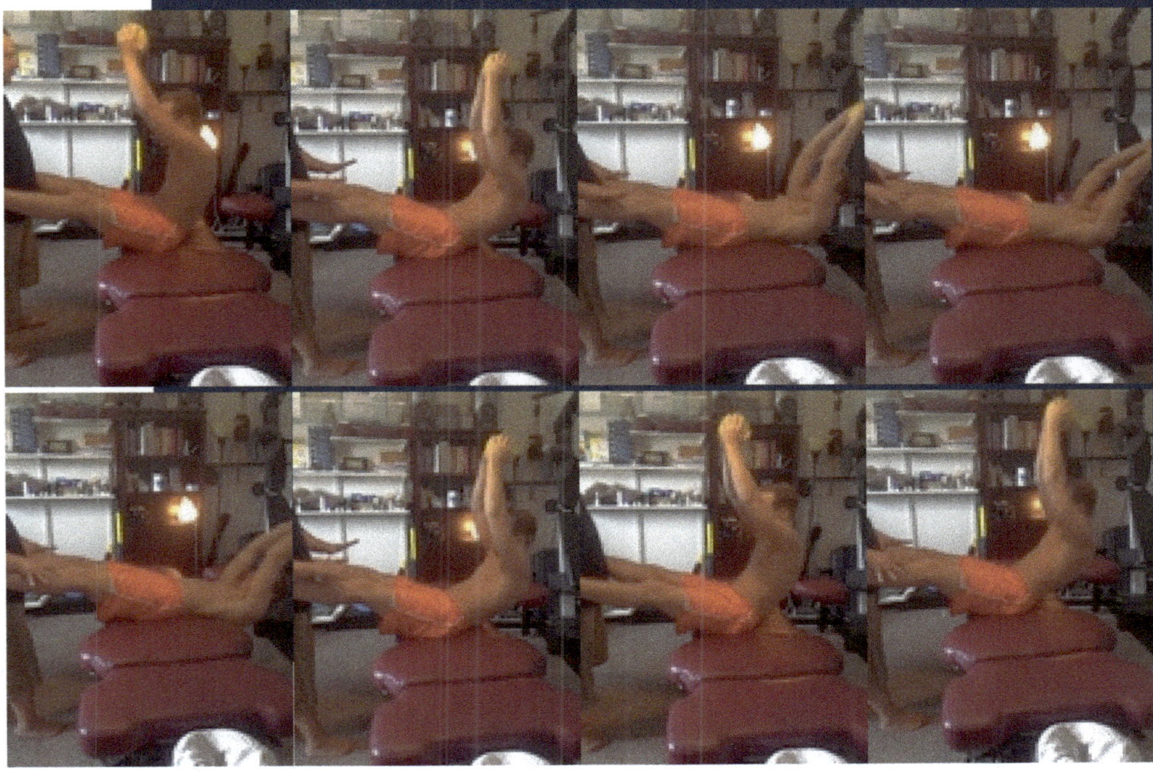

This is a more advanced exercise. Feet are wrapped around therapist squeezing while client has a weighted ball between hands also squeezing while doing a controlled crunch. One of the unique aspects of this is that sitting on a table like this challenges client's balancers while simultaneously engaging multiple muscle groups. Client is getting a great stretch throughout upper body while engaging multiple muscle groups at the same time. This is much

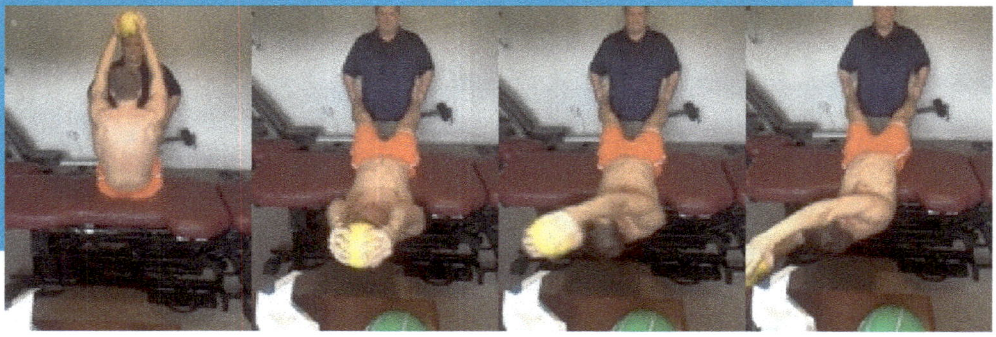

This is the same concept as before; however, we are going straight down and then side to side before coming back up. Now we are really starting to get oblique as well as stretching and training the rib cage, shoulder blades, deltoids, and upper and mid traps.

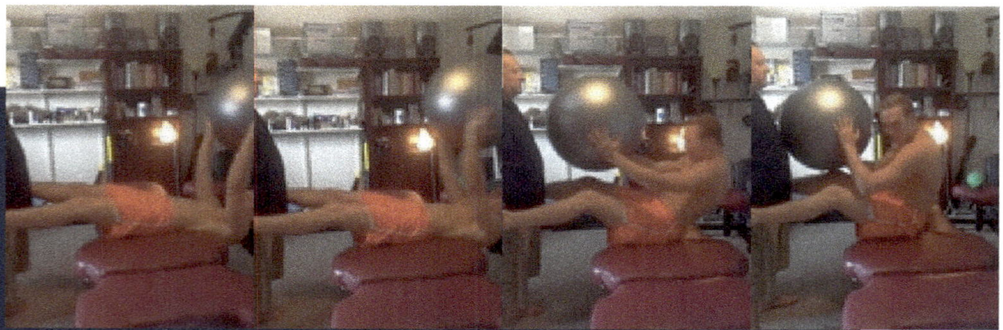

Changing the size of the ball will alter the muscle angles thereby engaging a different set of muscle fibers. Also, in this case, squeezing against a yoga ball like this versus a solid ball engages your stabilizers. You will find that your client's muscles will shake and vibrate more - thus increasing muscle endurance the harder they squeeze.

IN SUMMARY

Not only do we work the area in question such as shoulders, but we also work all of the surrounding musculature.

> *"The body does not move in isolated patterns during natural motion activities, so why train that way?"*
>
> **Ari Gronich, The Performance Therapist**

DISCUSSION:

1. Which muscle groups are involved in a free form dip between parallel bars?

____

2. Which muscle groups are involved in a seated, down press on a machine?

____

3. List the effects in the body when muscles begin to shake?

____

____

____

ANSWERS:

1. TRICEPS, CHEST SHOULDERS, THEN CORE 2. TRICEPS, LOWER CHEST, SHOULDERS, SOME CORE 3. MORE FIBERS FIRING, LYMPHATIC BENEFIT PUMPING TOXINS OUT OF MUSCLES, BALANCER MUSCLE BECOME INVOLVED IN THE ACTION, INCREASES BLOOD FLOW, DECREASES LACTIC ACID

THROUGHOUT TODAY, WHAT IS THE SINGLE MOST IMPORTANT STRATEGY YOU GOT THAT WILL ADD TO YOUR PRACTICE TOMORROW?

THE PERFORMANCE THERAPIST CERTIFICATION

Master Education Program

Level II Training Manual

LEVEL II
PERFORMANCE THERAPIST CERTIFICATE: WHAT YOU WILL LEARN TODAY

PREREQUISITE: PERFORMANCE THERAPY ACADEMY LEVEL I

MODULE I
DURATION: 3 HOURS

Advanced Exercise for Rehabilitation and Injury Prevention

This is an advanced extension of Modules 2 and 3 from Level I.

In our fast-paced lifestyle, it is easy to become distracted – from driving (or walking) while texting to going to the gym and working out too fast and too hard so that we can get home in time for the latest show. We trip and fall; we bump and scrape; we rip and shred our bodies.

Training for injury prevention and rehabilitation will give you an edge with the myriad of clients that come in with a variety of problems. From low back pain to shoulder injuries and more, no one is immune.

In this module you will spend time experiencing and facilitating non-impact training methods that not only build muscle strength, leverage, flexibility, and endurance but also serve to help prevent future injuries from occurring and also rehabilitate current and acute injuries. Many of these injuries become chronic and are then compensated for by the client creating other imbalances and conditions that need to be taken into consideration.

This will be a hands-on experience that will get your mind thinking creatively about how to address clients in a way you may not have thought about before.

An offshoot benefit of this module is that once you master it you will have the opportunity to get a wide variety of referrals from the medical world – clients who have been in auto accidents, or had workers comp or slip-and-fall injuries, recent surgery, and more.

MODULE II
DURATION: 3 HOURS

Program Design/Development/Management

With the uniqueness of each individual and the wide array of options we have, people want, and should be given, a treatment plan specific to them. One-size-fits-all training is obsolete and ineffective.

This module will introduce you to methods so that you (a) recognize each person's physical and mental starting place, (b) develop an individualized program, and (c) progress a client through a program and/or modify the program to adapt to the client's needs as they change. This may be a transformation in the way you view the intake process and how you then choose to work with your clients.

We will be creating programs based on several scenarios. You will be teamed up with a partner to go through the client history and develop protocols and programs that address all needs of the client as an individual.

MODULE III
DURATION: 2 HOURS

Introduction to Creating the Mindset of Change

How do we think? How do we feel? What are the blocks that hold us back from living the life we truly desire? Everyone is different and treating-every-client-the-same mentalities no longer work with clients. How then do we deliver to them the mindset to succeed?

This module is not just about how we think when treating our clients, but it's also about the markers that we look at for developing programs that help them get healthy. We will touch on everything from detoxification and brain chemistry to meditation and taking the best elements from all healing modalities to improve the outcomes for our clients. This is a chance to shift paradigms and wake up to the future of medicine and lifestyle changes.

We will focus on how to deliver the mindset of change to your clients so that you provide them the necessary ammunition to get beyond the blocks that hold them back from living to their full potential. Whether you are a personal trainer who always needs to motivate your clients into action or a doctor or nutritionist or therapist who is working hard to keep your patients compliant with their program, this is the section that will begin your journey into the minds and hearts of your clients.

All the knowledge in the world means nothing without the inner tools to make it last and keep it up for life. This course will teach you how to change your clients' lives and keep them inspiring their friends and family in the process.

LEVEL II: MODULE I

ADVANCED EXERCISE FOR REHABILITATION AND INJURY PREVENTION

MODULE I:
ADVANCED EXERCISE FOR REHABILITATION AND INJURY PREVENTION

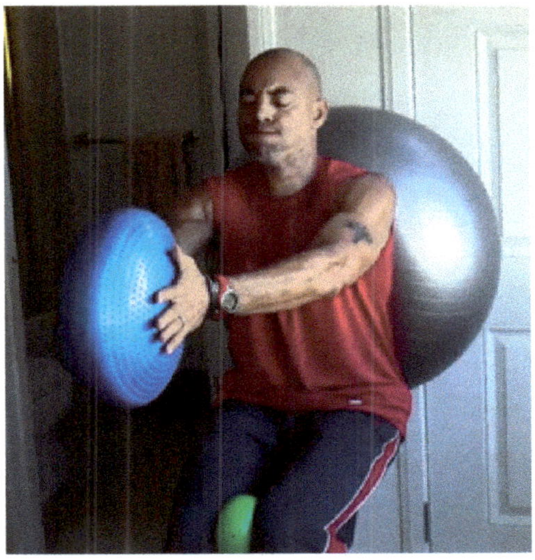

Dominique Arnold "PTA Advanced Squat"

Training for shape or weight loss or gain is different from training for either rehabilitation or for prevention of future injuries. Bodybuilders are notorious for their large muscles and shape; however, they are not well known for raw power. In fact, those that compete in lifting competitions rarely look much like the bodybuilding competitors. We must design unique training practices to address the differences in body types and goals that each client may have.

> *"There are principles in command for every style of training. When we go outside of these principles, there is a chance of counteracting the effectiveness and falling short of the goals."*
>
> **Ari Gronich, The Performance Therapist**

Whether training someone for competition bodybuilding or training them for injury prevention and rehabilitation, keeping the principles of training in mind will help guide your programs and keep you and your clients on track.

PRINCIPLES OF EXERCISES DEVELOPED FOR REHABILITATION AND INJURY PREVENTION:

- Train slowly, and engage as much muscle fiber into action as possible with every movement.
- Non-Impact and Low-Impact training will decrease the jarring on joints and bones.
- Flexibility training will engage your ligaments and tendons to produce long levers and a deep ROM.
- Every exercise engages the core and stabilizing muscles.
- With injury-specific areas, we bring blood flow and stress to damaged tissue with NO impact.
- Every angle is paid attention to, thereby exercising the body through full ROM; emphasize finding and targeting the weakest areas of the body and strengthening them.
- Warm up the body with sauna, spa, bath, hot towels, massage, light cardio, light stretching, walking, etc.
- Use body weight exercises with progressions before weight lifting equipment or machines.

Utilizing these basic principles, you will be developing exercises and training protocols that cater to this underserved community of injured clients.

INTERACTIVE DRILL

SCENARIO – LONG DISTANCE CYCLER

Client walks into your studio. You observe a slight limp on the right leg; the hips are square, but the left shoulder is slightly higher than the right, and the client seems to have some difficulty turning his head. Client appears to be between late 40s to early 50s and in relatively good shape.

During the intake process you learn that the client is 52 years old, has had 2 surgeries on right knee, and has been told he has about 15% cartilage remaining so is close to bone on bone. Current complaint is: either turned head wrong or slept wrong, not sure, but now can hardly twist left to right and is having spasms down upper spine and shoulder blades mostly on the left side.

Client wants to get out of immediate pain but also has a goal. It is a 150-mile bike ride, with a 5000 elevation climb starting at altitude. Has done the ride prior at 12.5 average mph. At altitude was suffering from breathing issues, and throughout the ride was cramping up. Now, 10 years later, wants to ride the same course and improve the numbers.

In this scenario, we will progress the client from Day 1 through a 6-month training process that will prepare him to beat the previous time while also eliminating all issues of the ride. Oh, by the way, client cannot get on a bike for the first 3 months. We will be shifting habits and patterns and don't want client to fall back into old imbalances before body is ready for the activity.

Team up with a partner and choose an A and a B

A – Client
B – Trainer

Week 1

Eliminate spasm in neck and begin to relax upper back and shoulders; start slow with beginning exercises on right knee.

Tx – Treatment Plan

3 days a week for the first 4 weeks; TOTAL REST ON DAYS OFF

EXERCISES

NECK EXERCISES

For trainers use a medium length thin towel; for massage therapists, use your hands and/or a towel or pillow case.

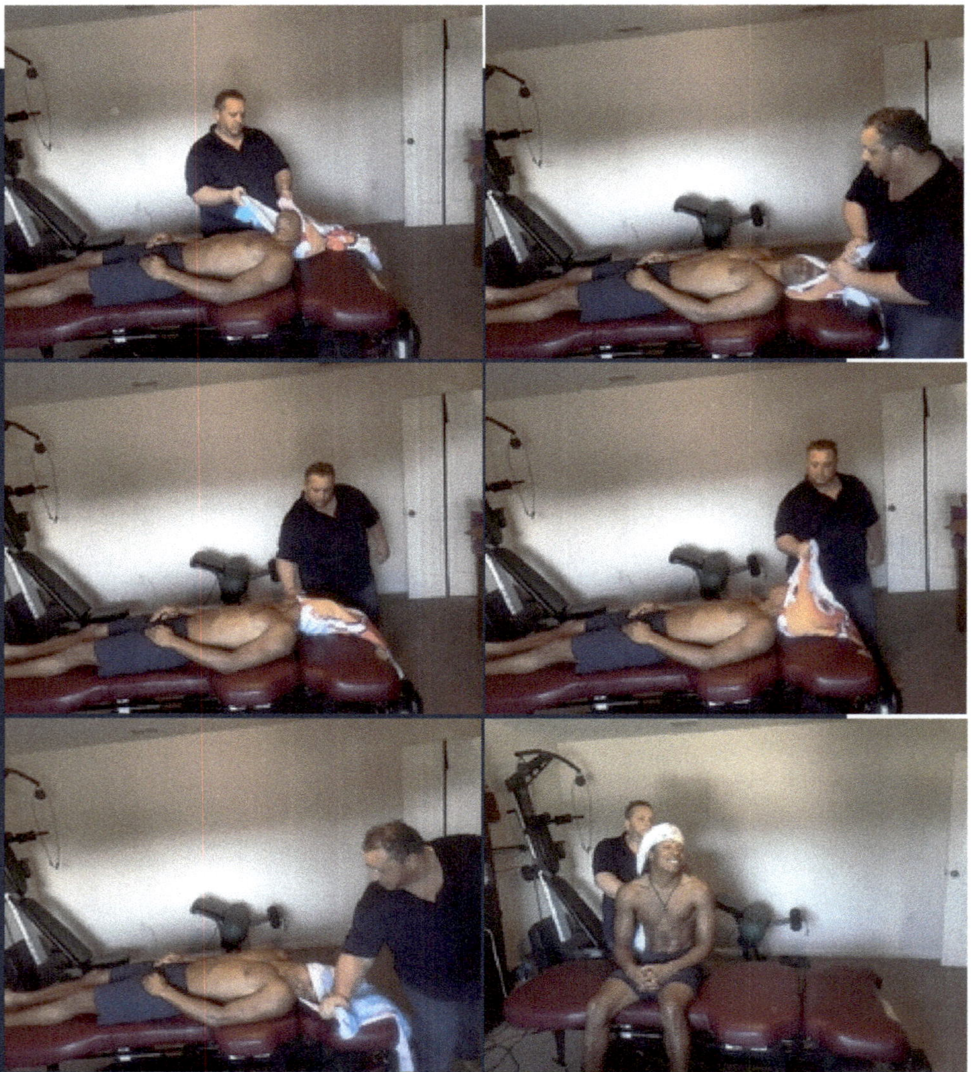

Place a towel under the occipital ridge. Stretching at every possible angle. When you get to the extent of the Range of Motion, have the client resist against the pull of the towel. These exercises will not only stretch the attachments of the neck, but also will exercise the musculature - including upper trapezius, shoulders, and core. In the last frame on the page we have seated the client and have placed the towel around his forehead. He is resisting the motion in multiple directions. The resistance that you, as a Performance Therapist, are providing is in direct correlation to the power of the client.

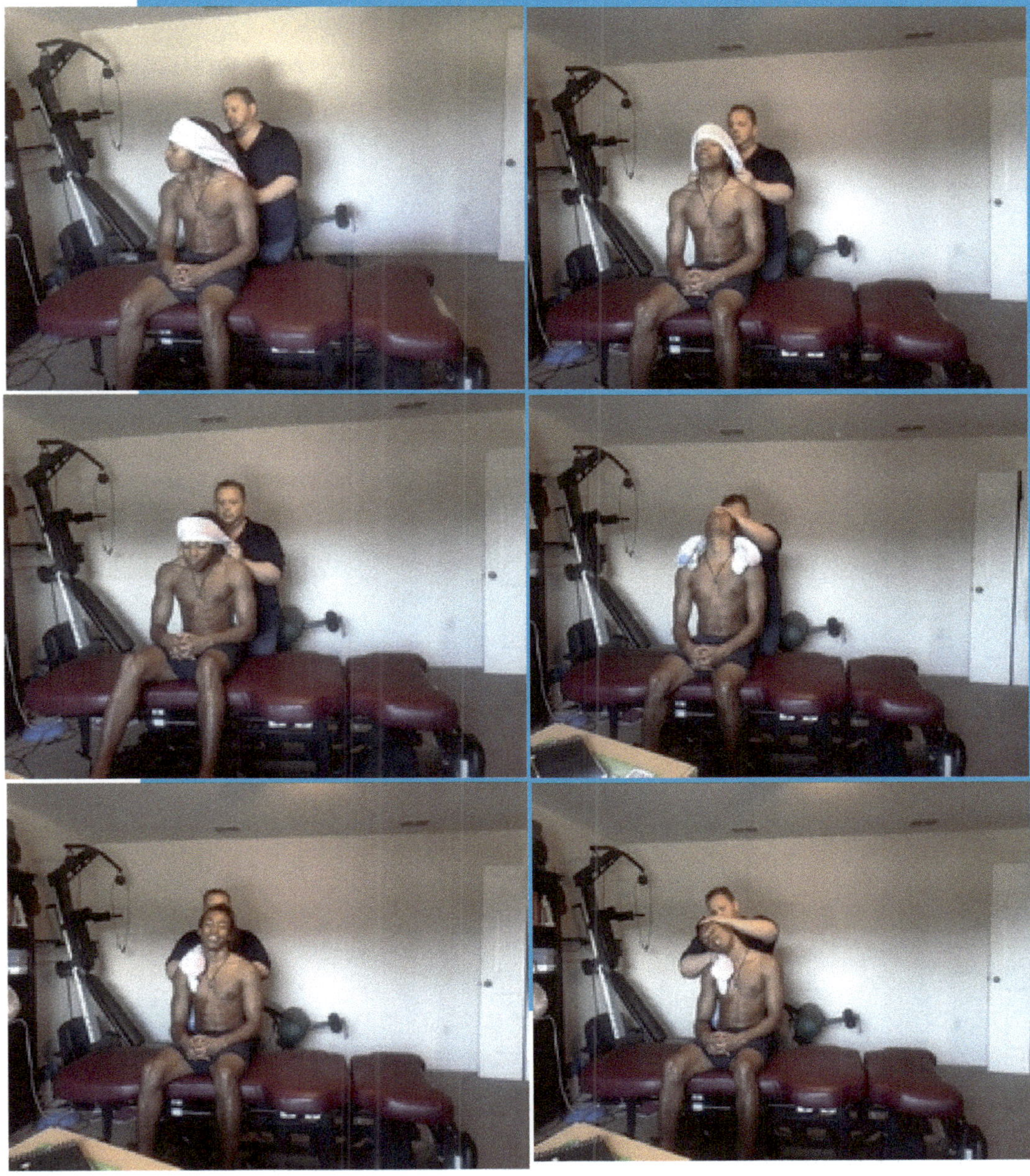

These multi-directional stretches with resistance will not only help fatigue the muscle and alleviate cramping, but they will also add ROM and power giving them more resistance to future injury. In the last three frames on this page, the towel is bundled or rolled up and placed at the back of the neck or on the shoulders and the client is squeezing the towel in between either the neck and back or neck and shoulder. Again, this kind of resistance will both add to the ROM and power felt by the client as well as increase muscle suppleness and comfort. When finished, your client will not only feel like he has had a great workout, but he should also feel pretty loose and relaxed.

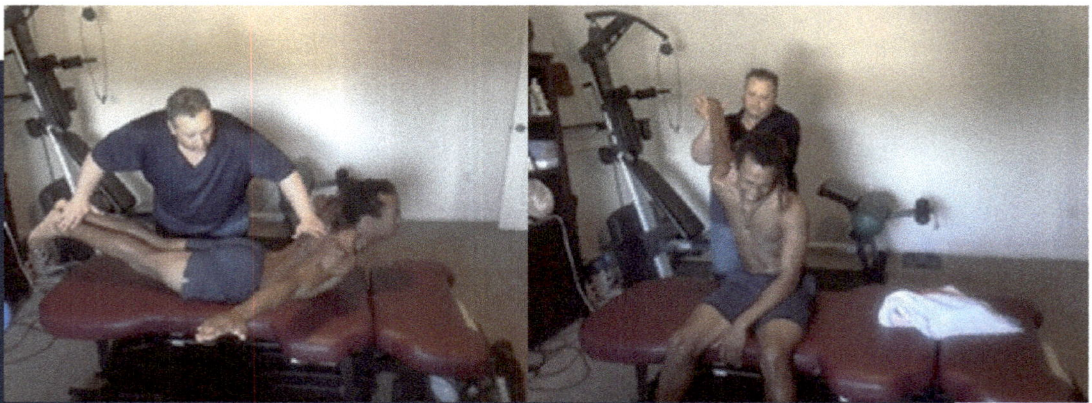

In the superman pose on the left, client is resisting both at legs and upper body. He is squeezing glutes, hamstrings, and core muscles throughout low back, trapezius, and more. Shoulders can move from the sides to straighten out in front for multiple angles and directions which will strengthen and lengthen the shoulder joints. In the seated position on the right, client is resisting down and then up. At the wrist we slowly guide his arm to the top of his ROM. That is where resistance will begin. Allow him to move through the entire range of motion for optimum effect.

Weeks 2 – 4

Get the body moving one joint after another. Range of Motion and Stability Focused.

THERAPIST/TRAINER GUIDED ON FLOOR OR TREATMENT TABLE OR BENCH: FOOT, KNEE, HIP ROTATION

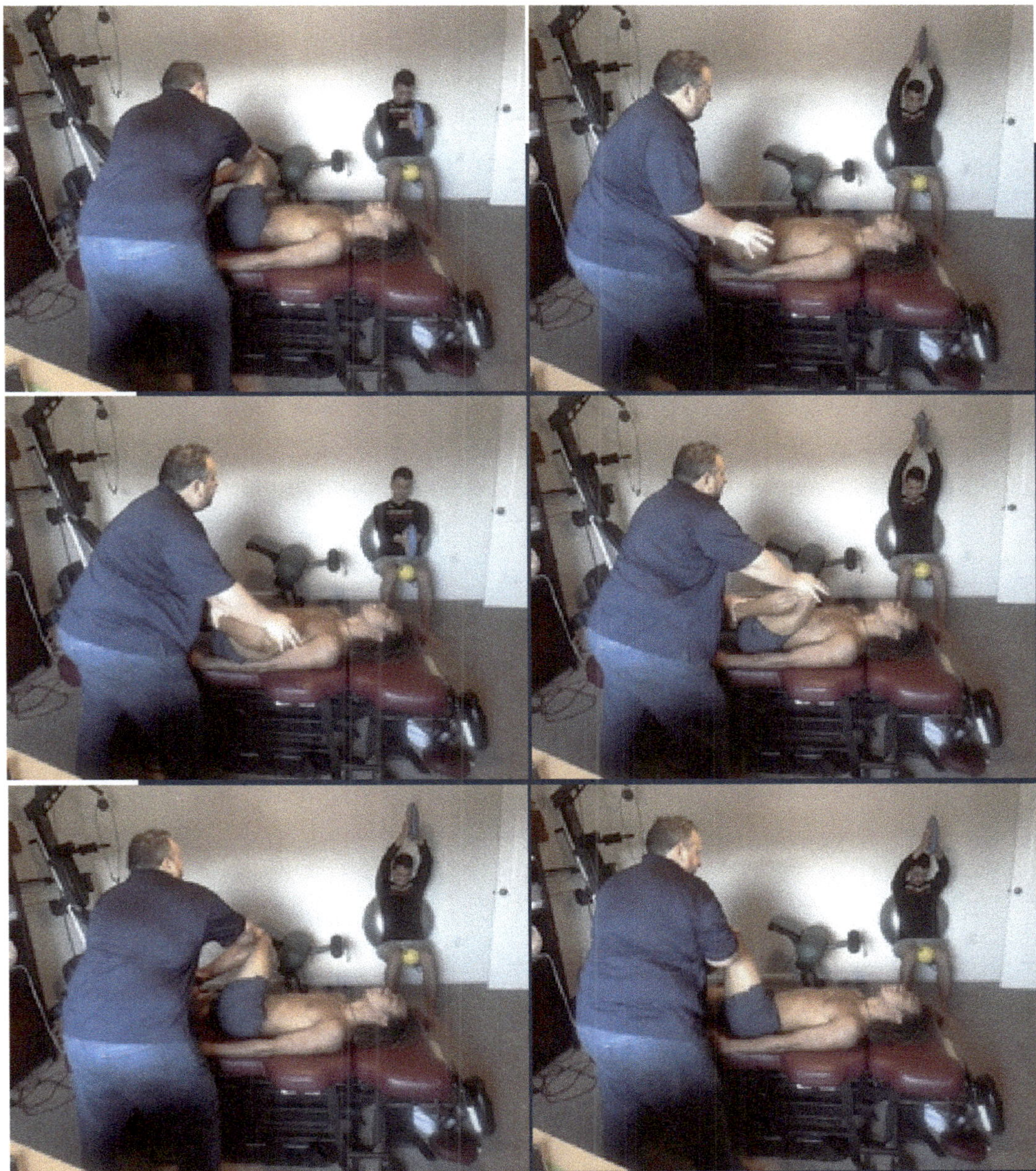

These frames depict trainer mobilization of client. That means the client is simply lying in position while the Performance Therapist does all of the work. Rotations at every angle; knee toward opposite side of body, and then swing around extending knee out stretching groin, then moving up to chest and swinging around the entire ROM of the hip joint. Most people are tight when moving across the point of the belly with the knee. This is indicative of tight psoas muscle. Try to stabilize the upper pelvis and hip to maximize the stretching of the psoas.

THERAPIST/TRAINER GUIDED EITHER ON FLOOR OR A TREATMENT TABLE OR BENCH: SHOULDER AND UPPER BODY ROTATIONS

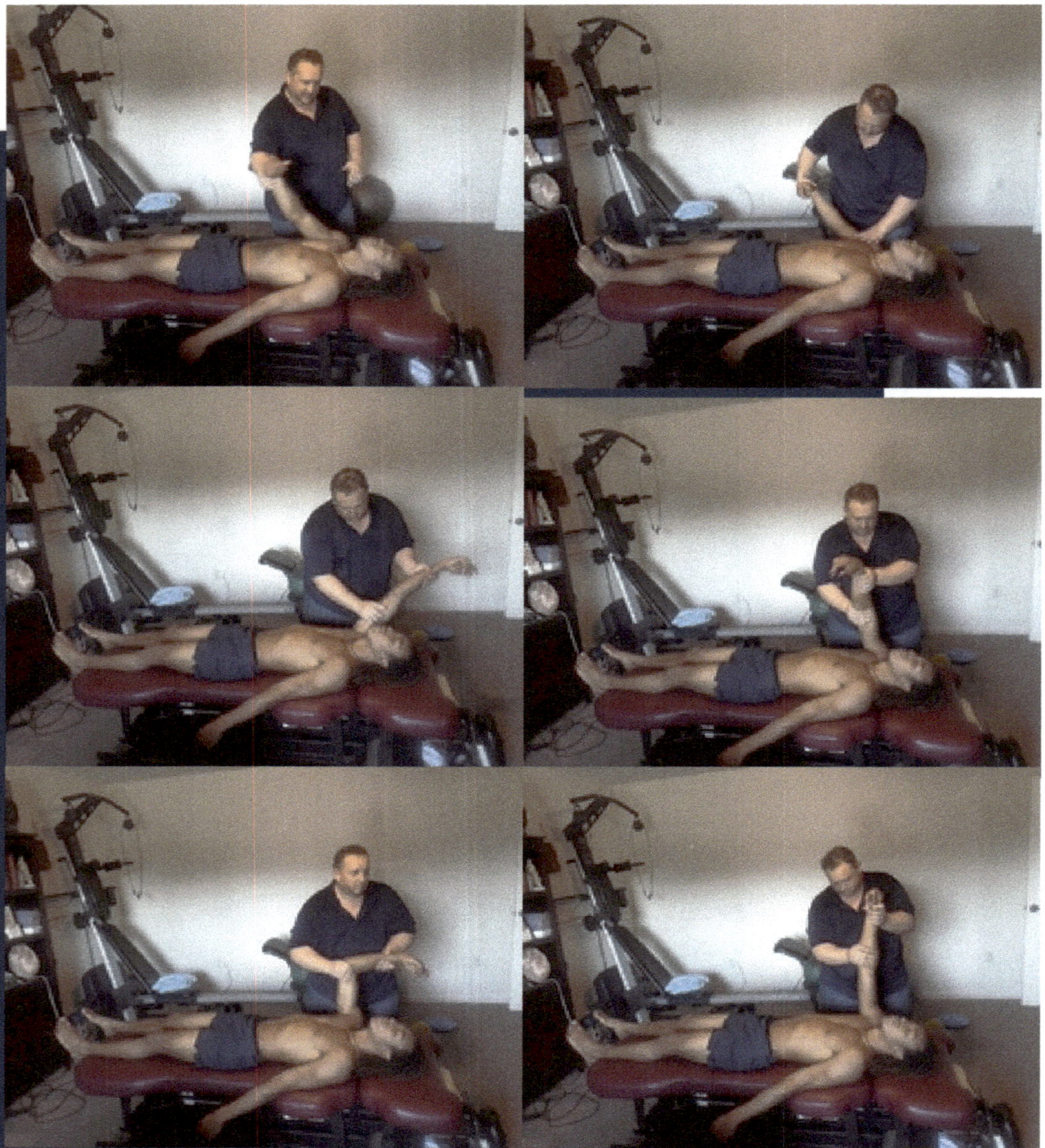

Supine position while holding wrist: guide the shoulder throughout the ROM. Rotate the hand from outward to inward in order to get every angle possible. Important point to note: when mobilizing a joint, make sure client is NOT resisting your movement. Pay attention because when resistance occurs, it could be an injury or simply a point in which the ROM is limited - and those are areas to work on further and investigate more closely.

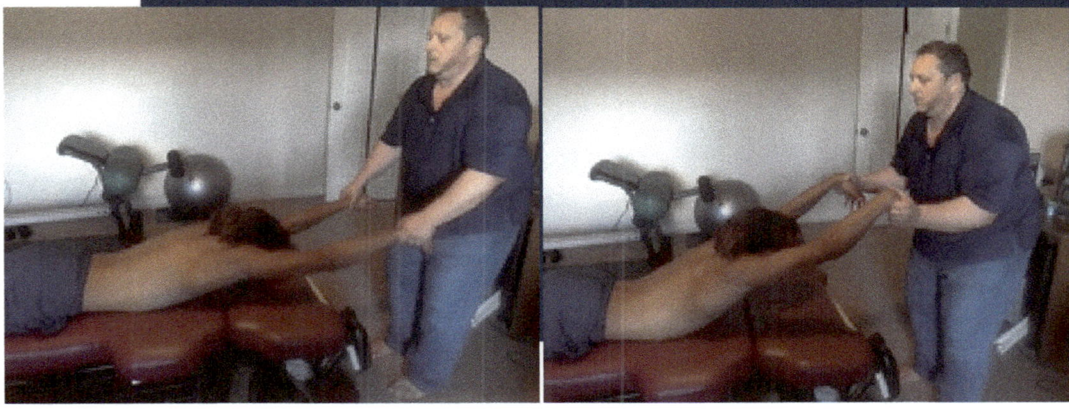

In the first frame, the Performance Therapist is simply providing traction for the upper body by getting a good grip and leaning back. You can even move side to side to open up the obliques as well as latissimus muscles.

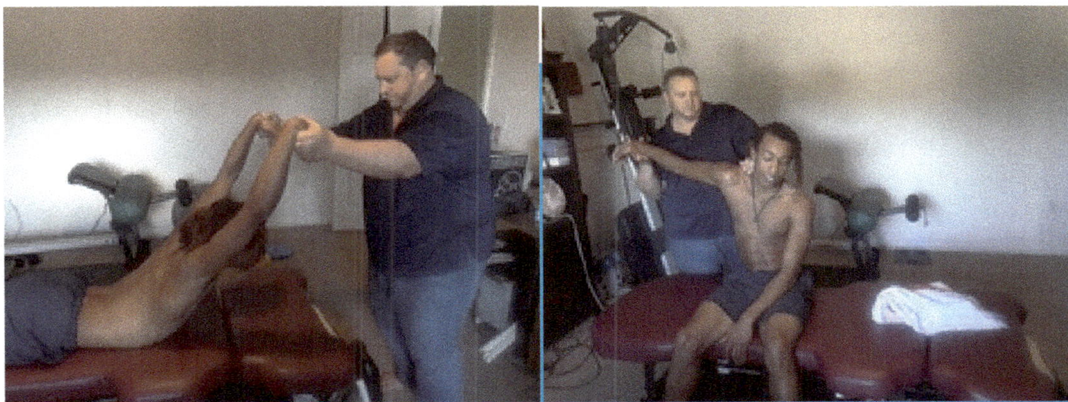

The frame on the left uses the leverage of the hand to wrist grip and raises the upper body off the table allowing for gravity to pull down, thus creating an intense stretch for the upper front of the body.

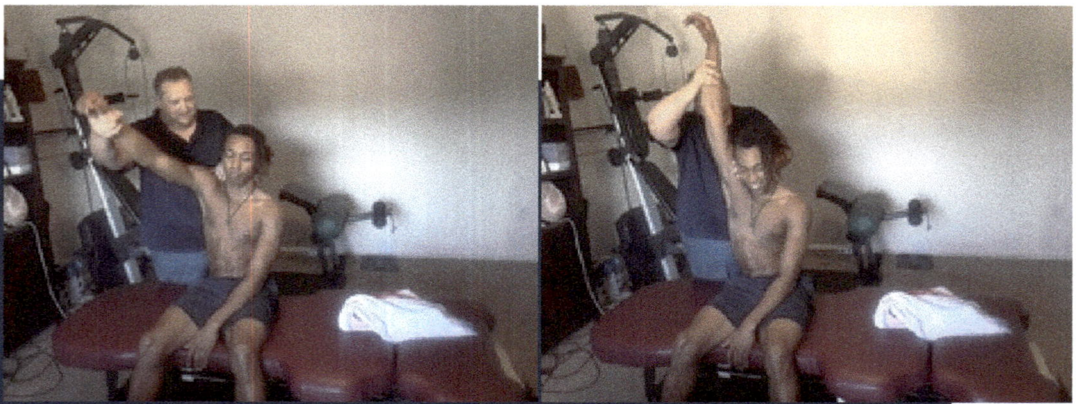

These last 4 frames depict the rotation and mobilization of shoulders through neck. Isolate the shoulder by placing pressure on the upper traps, and relax that pressure when you want to stretch the entire muscle chain.

Weeks 5 – 12

Strength and Endurance Focus

Tx

3 days a week in office
1 day a week stretching on client's own; TOTAL REST ON DAYS OFF.

PTA (PERFORMANCE THERAPY ACADEMY) LEG LIFTS: VARIOUS POSITIONS AND EXERCISES

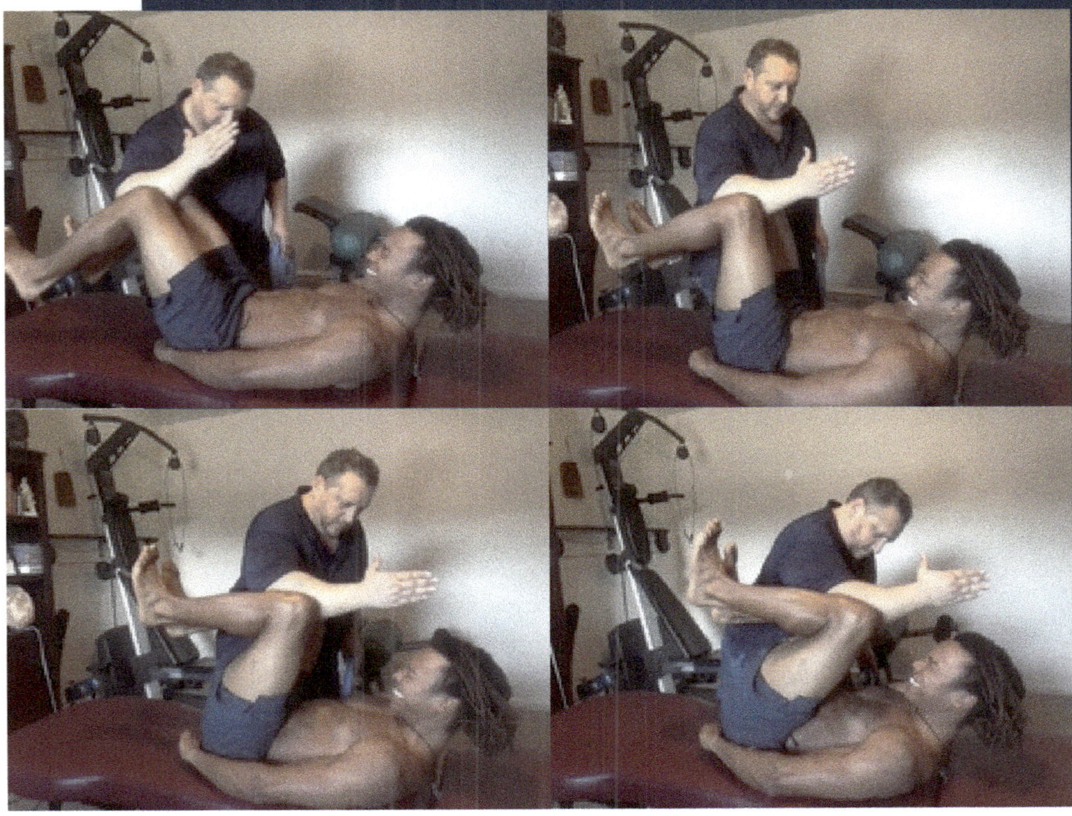

The four frames above depict a great full body workout. Starting from the leg lift perspective, with knees bent, have client squeeze your arm. While the knees are squeezing, the Performance Therapist is pushing up towards the chest. Now we are working the inner thighs, psoas, quads, hamstrings, and even the calf muscles will engage in the activity to resist moving upwards. Core muscles, upper stomach, abs, chest, and also the shoulders tend to get involved. Remember to reverse the motion and have the client resist downward movement toward the floor, but only after holding a sustained squeeze at the peak of client's ROM towards head.

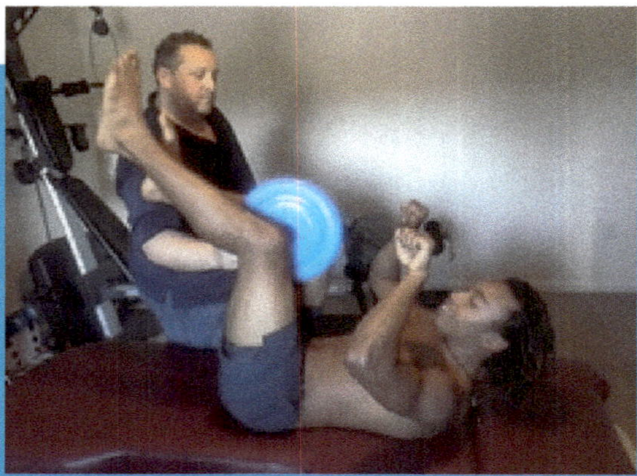

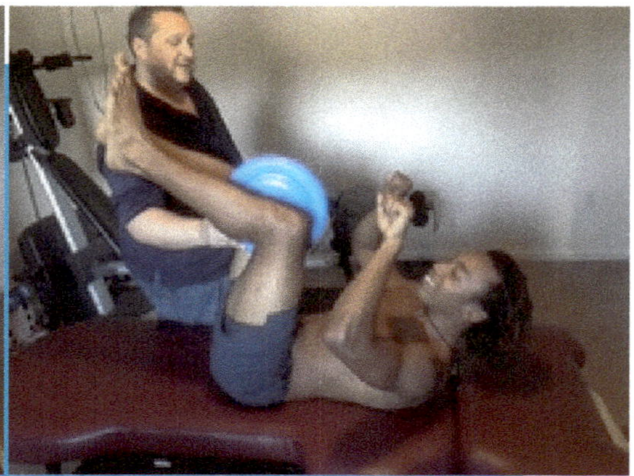

These two frames above provide both an evaluation as well as a training possibility. Place a thin disc approximately the size of a bicycle bar between the client's knees. Next have them peddle as though on a bicycle. Arms are in handlebar position and upper back is slightly elevated off the table.

As an evaluation process, watch to see if the hips and knees are rotating towards the outside. If the outer hip and IT band are tight, they will pull the knee out of the plane. This will be an area to focus on and balance inner thigh strength with. Having balanced strength in the abductors and adductors will shave time off the ride while also reducing fatigue and cramping. When the balance is regular, you can use this exercise for endurance and speed drills going from resistance to simulate climbing to sprinting on the flats and relaxed pedaling in the downgrades.

PTA SHOULDER AND FOREARM TRAINING

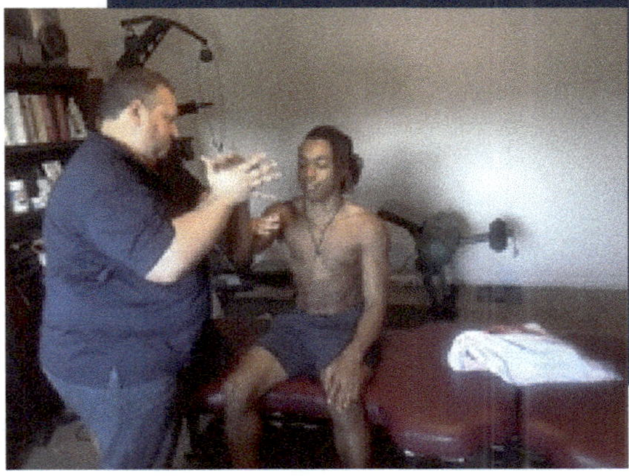

Place your hand at the crease of the client's hand.

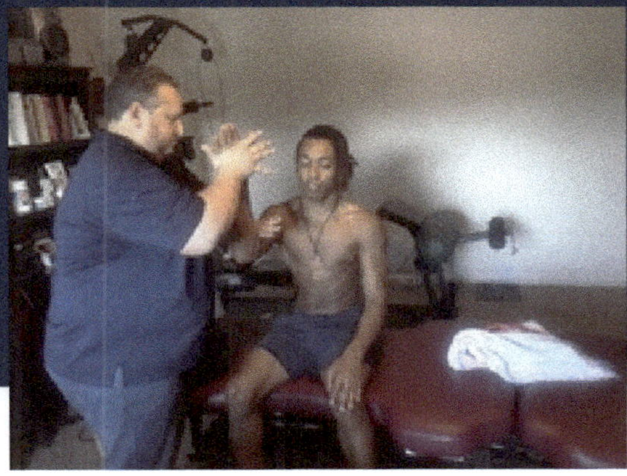

Stabilize the elbow and have client straighten the elbow.

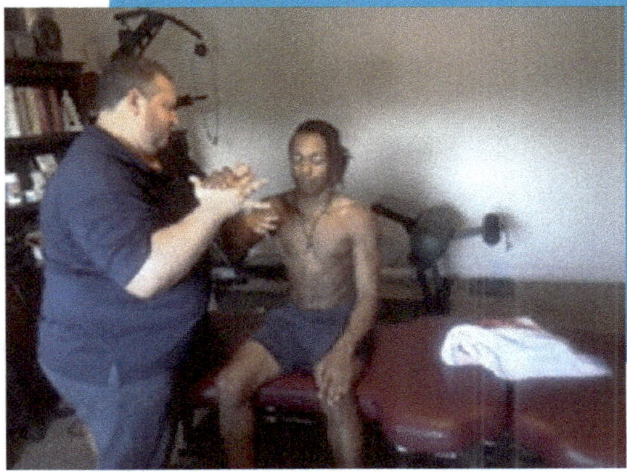

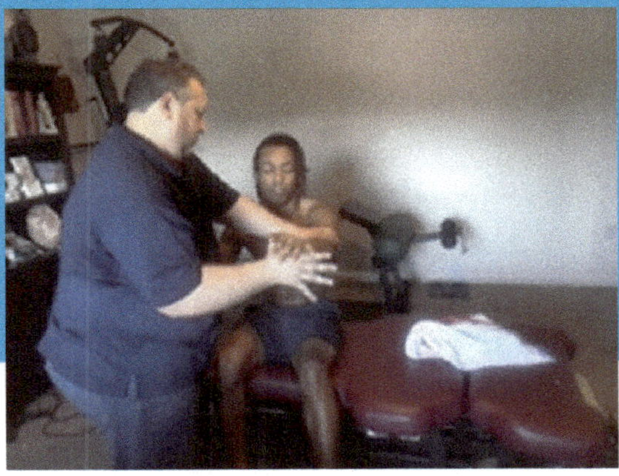

There are variations of this exercise with hand rotated throughout ROM. Great forearm and tricep exercise. Adds ROM and strengthens the elbow joint. Multiple Directions of Resistance required to get 360° effect.

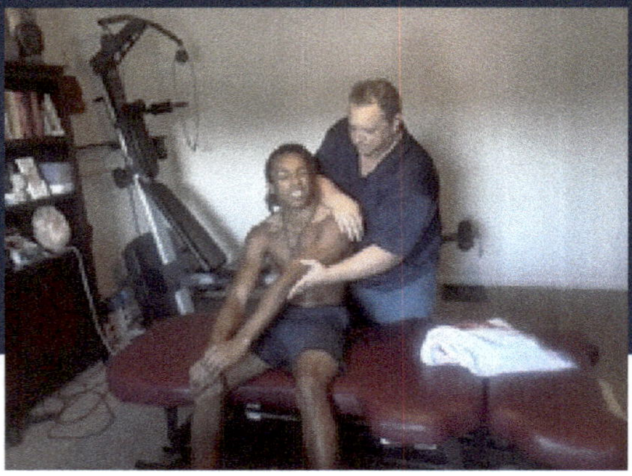

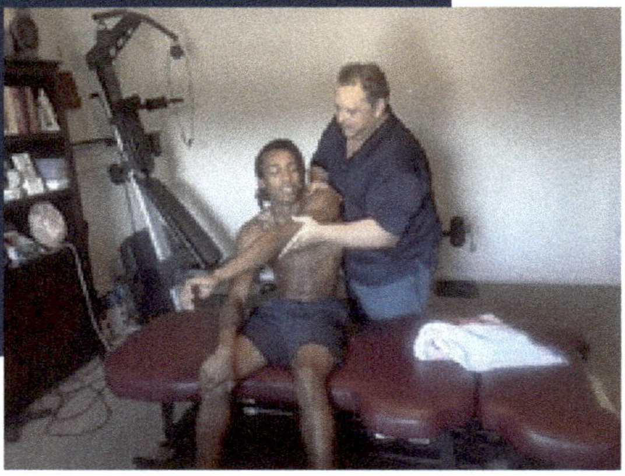

Using forearm, stabilize the shoulder from raising up as you place arm across the body. Once at the extent of ROM, have the client resist towards the outside. This should be done all the way through the ROM and with hand rotated each time in a different position. Hand can be up then down, then pinkie up, and then thumb up, etc.

Weeks 13 – 18

Speed and Endurance Focus – Back on the bike again

Tx

2 days a week in office – 1 day a week stretching on client's own - 1 day on bike with trainer – 1 day on bike on client's own; TOTAL REST ON DAYS OFF

EXERCISES

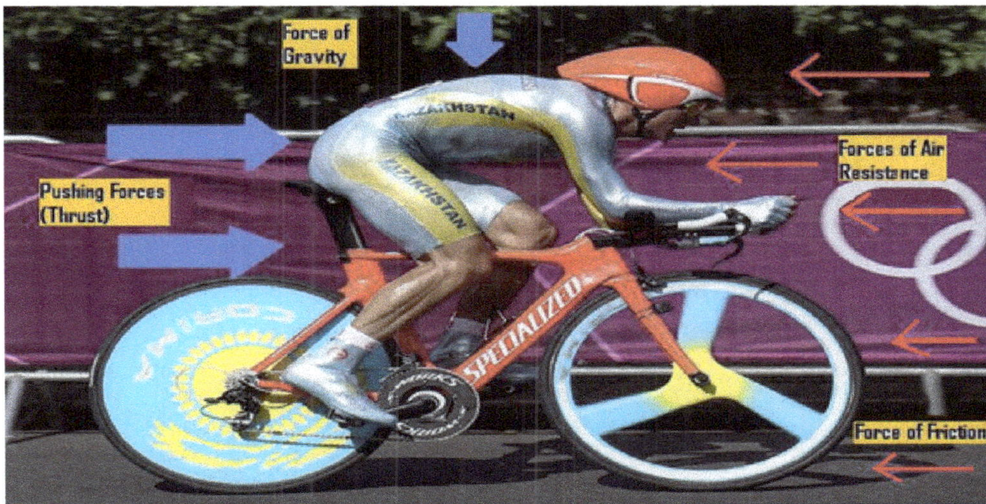

At home or with mobile trainer.

Hill Sprints if a gym bike elevation climb...Client is going to sprint uphill on his bike. The condition of client will determine what the hill grade will be. As we progress, the hill grade will steepen as well. Rest period will be a coast down the hill and then just as quickly sprinting back up the hill. Remember this is a sprint, not a marathon, so keep the pace moving. If you live in a town that is FLAT, sprint against the wind, put the gears on the most resistance, and possibly wear an altitude training mask.

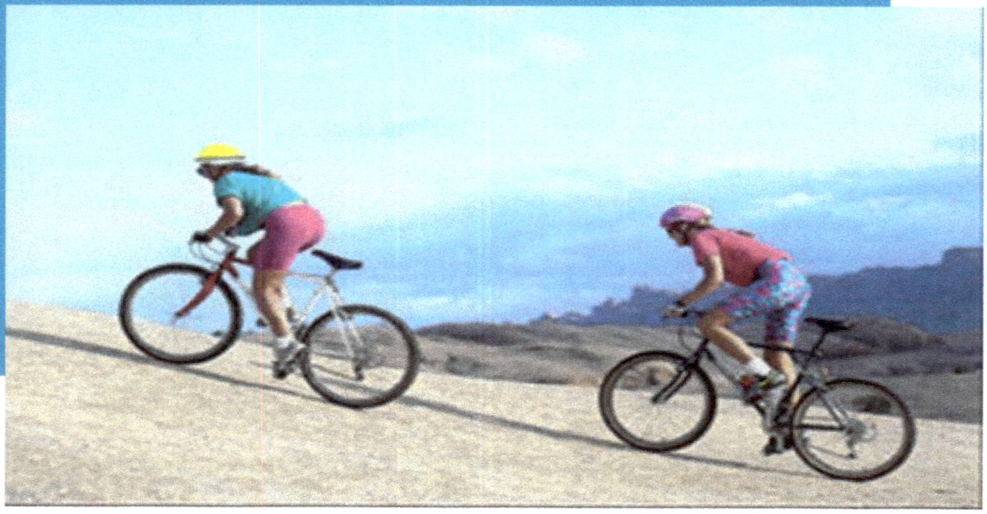

Velocity Enhanced Resistance Training

Add resistance and speed or pressure. The harder you go, an equal level of resistance will occur. (For example, when swimming, the harder you kick, the more the water resists you. The lighter you kick, the easier for your leg to move through water.)

This level of resistance will challenge the kinetic chain in a way that builds tremendous endurance, speed, and agility as well as increasing core strength and stability - all needed to accomplish the main goal.

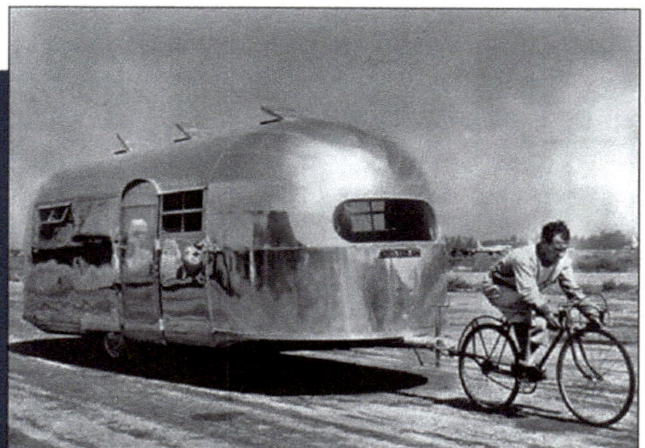

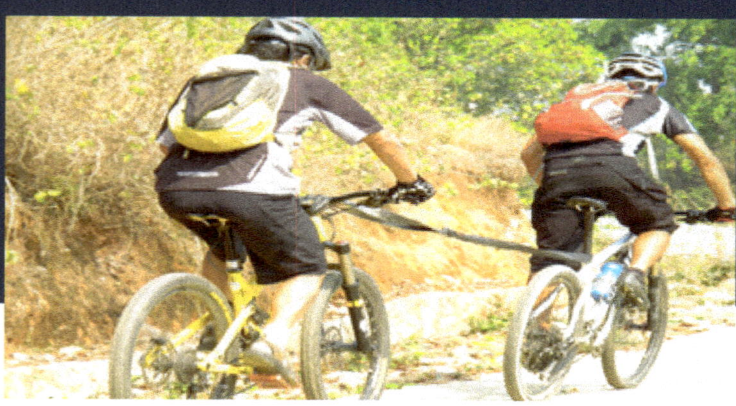

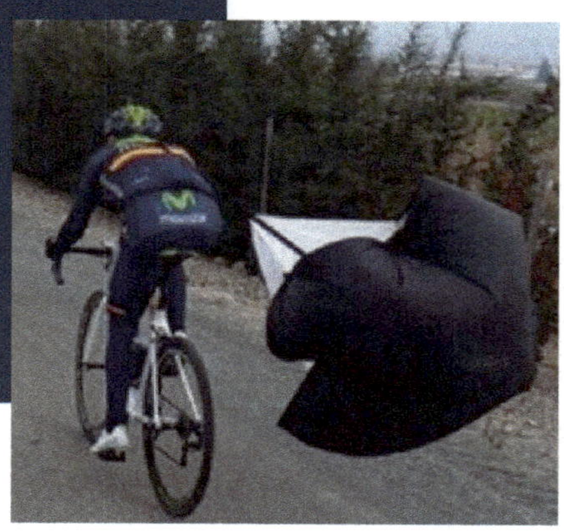

DRILL STYLE EXERCISES TO CHALLENGE THE MUSCLES' ENDURANCE AND STRENGTH WHILE PICKING UP SPEED. THESE EXERCISES ARE SPEED PLUS RESISTANCE IN NATURE AND CAN BE INNOVATED ON THE SPOT.

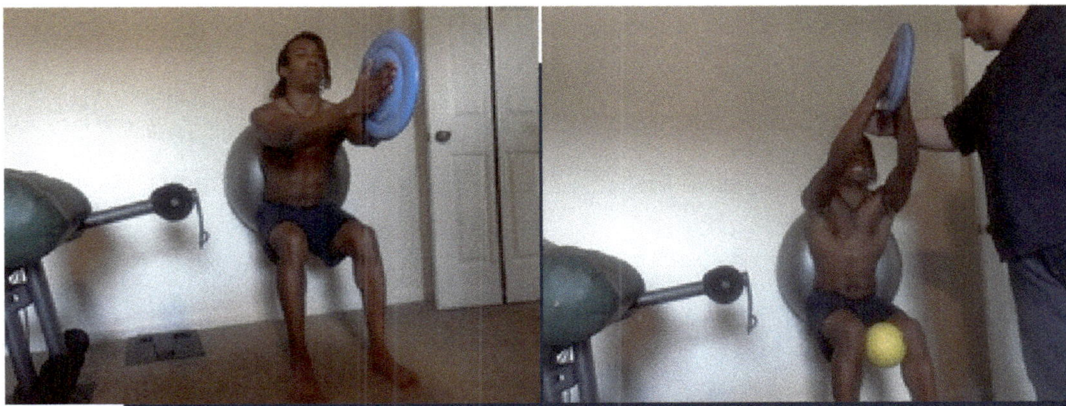

A PTA squat works the body on multiple planes and in multiple directions. We utilize an exercise ball at the back to maintain proper back support; however, we get the added benefit of challenging stability since client is not on a solid wall. In frame two you can see a progression of this movement adding a weighted ball between the knees.

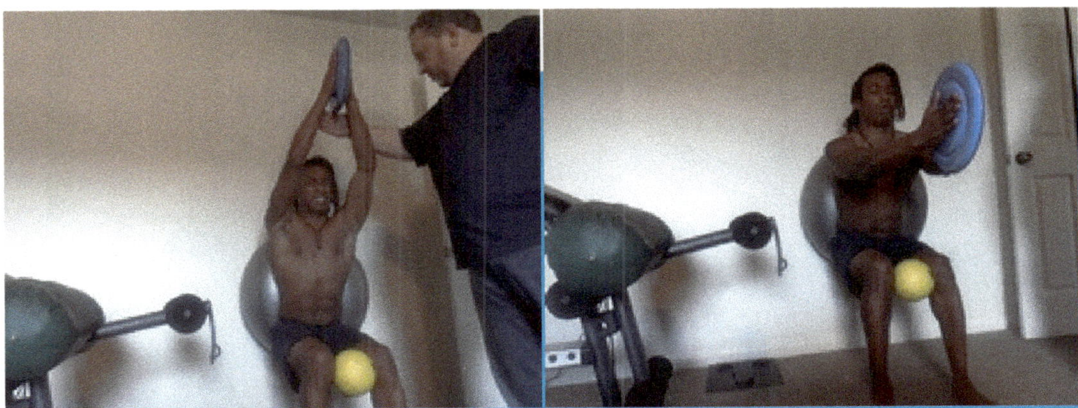

Squeeze on the ball while maintaining a seated position, with client pushing his feet forward into the floor while back is pushing up against the ball into the wall. Now, with the disc between his arms, have him squeeze tightly and move through the ROM of his shoulders from high to low and back up again!

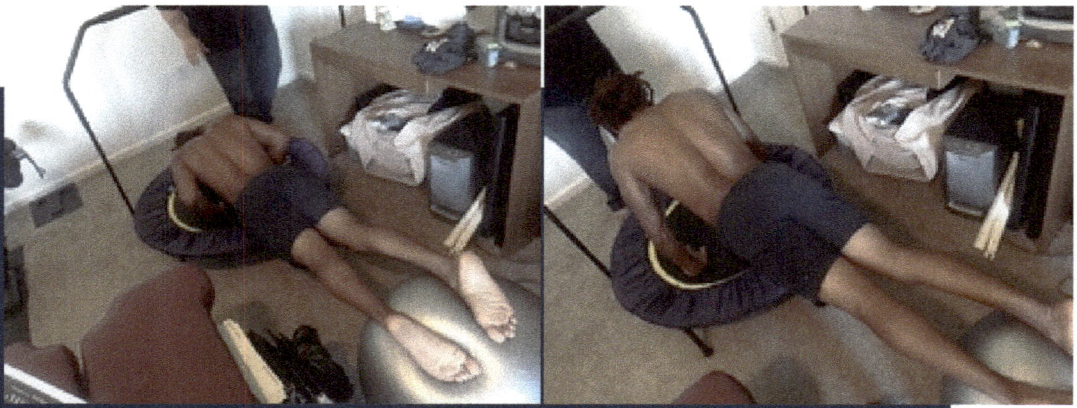

In the first frame client is in a down pushup position. With micro pushes he is bouncing slightly pushing down into the trampoline's netting. This causes a series of contractions that act to really strengthen the elbow joint as well as trapezius and at the same time engages the core muscles. Placing feet on the ball adds to the use of stabilizing muscles throughout the body. Next frame is a general pushup starting position. Same micro pushes into the trampoline netting. Continue this throughout the elbows' entire ROM.

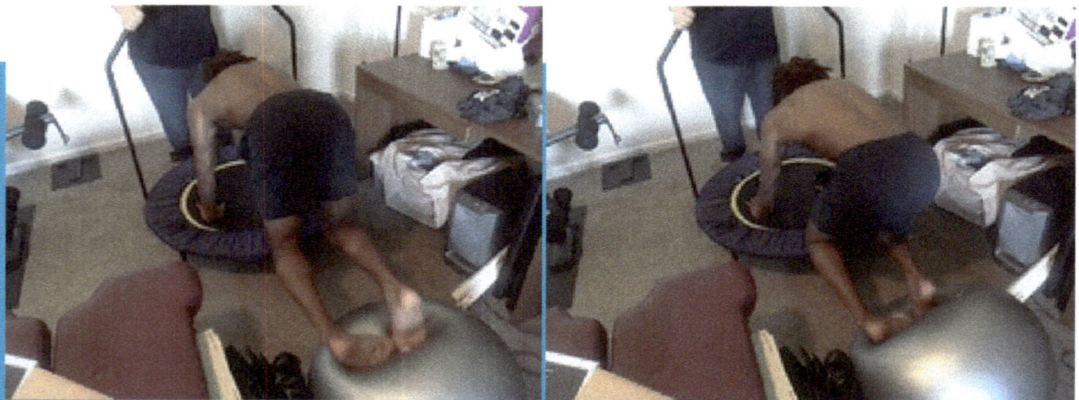

From the pushup positions client will now draw his feet close to his body with his knees as close to chest as possible throughout this ROM. This exercise works not only the quads and core but also the feet, forearms, shoulders, back muscles, and more. These will build muscle endurance, strength, and flexibility and provide the conditions for injury prevention.

Weeks 19 – 23

Return to basics. Make sure we are progressing to the end goal.

Tx

Based on Assessment

Be sure you have addressed everything that was on the challenge list. Check lungs and air intake. Start your client on keeping a log of cramping episodes and food so we can correlate the two if one directly has a causation effect.

We have six weeks to make sure that all goals are reached. Now is the time to check the numbers and vitals, correct any postural issues or muscular imbalances, etc.

Each week we repeat exercises based on assessments and add resistance such as sprinting uphill with a heavy backpack on, or even with a mini parachute, etc.

Week 24

- 7 days from the Big Ride – Go Hard. Train all out. Client will train with trainer in the morning, go for a half to three-quarter ride either 75 or 100 miles, and then come back and stretch out with trainer again (on ride day you will be going for another 50-75 miles so this will challenge stamina, endurance, and muscle ability.)
- 6 days from Big Ride - TOTAL REST
- 5 days from the Big Ride – Go Medium. Today will only be a 50 mile ride. Morning warmup at home followed by ride followed by a medium-intensity workout
- 4 days from Big Ride - TOTAL REST
- 3 days from the Big Ride – Go Soft. Today client will do an easy, leisurely 25 miles taking his time and checking out the scenery. Next will be a light training session to create mobility in all the joints. Joint mobility is key for the ride so the looser and more fluid we can get the joints, the better. Intake LOTS OF FLUIDS.
- 2 days from Big Ride - TOTAL REST
- Day 1 from the Big Ride – Meditation Day. Trainer can help create an audio of a guided meditation that the client could use throughout the day. Client will be lying down in his most comfortable chair at least 3-6 times during the day - and can even put the meditation on loop while he sleeps. This meditation will guide the client through the entire ride from how his body feels to the wind in his hair to the rumble of the road and the sweat on his brow. This is a meditation that describes what he has already done as he was doing it.

(I was going around the bend at mile 38, climbing at 5% grade. My muscles were warm and my shoulders felt strong as I pushed forth in front of two other riders. The wind was whipping through my hair and as I got to the top of the bend and my muscles were really feeling powerful, I saw the down grade and knew I was in for quite a ride.) Something along those lines.

- Day of the Big Ride – Wake up refreshed to a nice liter of water. Take a nice cold shower and put on some sweats. Run through a light resistance warm up with stretching with client's trainer. Take time to listen one more time to the meditation and then get on bike nice and relaxed and ready!

CONCLUSION
– A DAY OR TWO LATER

We go over the numbers and assess how well we did.

1. What were the results
(Met all the client's needs. Client increased average mph to 16; had zero breathing issues; zero cramping)

2. What elements led to this result?
(i.e. rest in between, varied program?)

3. What could be improved?
(Begin training sooner; set an actual goal number)

LEVEL II: MODULE II

PROGRAM DESIGN/ DEVELOPMENT/ MANAGEMENT

MODULE II:
PROGRAM DESIGN/ DEVELOPMENT/ MANAGEMENT

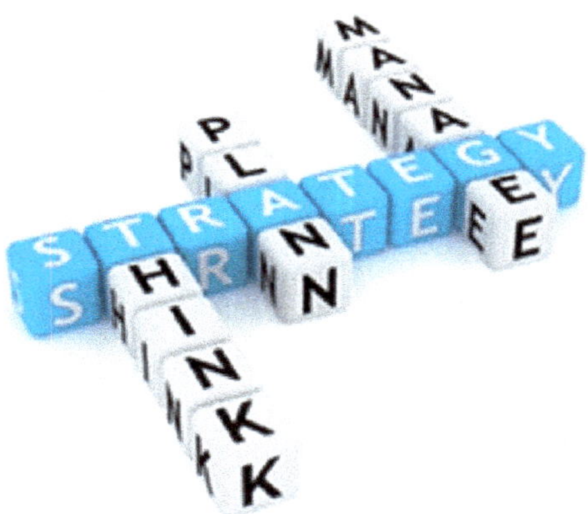

Being able to develop unique and individualized programs for clients will skyrocket your success. Due to the nature of developing programs like these, clients will be naturally drawn to you over the average cookie-cutter therapist.

In Module I we went through a possible scenario of training an athlete for a goal. That scenario could have been programmed in any one of a thousand different ways; however, programs must be designed with the end goal in mind while still taking into consideration the current state of the individual client. Being able to differentiate between a realistic goal and what might be a pie-in-the-sky goal is an important aspect of program development.

How do you think that kind of program development can help your business? Is it something you see yourself implementing? If yes, why?

In this module, we are going to delve into how you can begin developing programs utilizing exercises similar to those in Module I. This section is experiential in nature as it guides you in the creation process.

WHAT WE ARE LOOKING FOR IS WHETHER YOU HAVE BROUGHT THE KNOWLEDGE AND UNDERSTANDING FROM LEVEL I AND THE BEGINNING OF LEVEL II INTO HOW YOU THINK ABOUT A CLIENT.

There are indicators that an intake process identifies when developing a program. Having an in-depth intake process allows you to garner a sufficient level of information about the possible client to create the perfect individualized program. When developing a program, there are several key points to keep in mind.

SOME OF THE INDICATIONS TO LOOK FOR ARE:

SEVERITY OF THE CASE	Does the person coming in require a low, moderate, or high level of care?
MOTIVATION	Both current as well as long term motivation. Is this person ready to make the changes needed to go through a prescribed program?
CONTRAINDICATIONS	What are the things we simply cannot do with the client due to injuries, illnesses, mindsets, etc.?
GOALS AND EXPECTATIONS	How well can you measure and manage the goals and expectations of yourself and the client so that you maintain constant improvement in the long term and in a sustainable manner?
SUPPORT SYSTEM	What is the home and work life like and how much work will be required to gain the support of friends, family, co-workers, etc.?
TIME MANAGEMENT	Is the client willing to make the time needed a priority?

Sometimes it is best when developing a program to work backwards from the end goal. Work your way toward the present so that you have a goal-driven path to work from.

How can thinking in this way and being able to create a program like this benefit your practice?

INTERACTIVE EXERCISE

Team up into 2 or 3 (depending on count of the room)

I will present each group with a different scenario and you will create a 3-12-month program depending on what is necessary with that client based on the scenario.

(Hint: Refer to Module I – how can you take that information and utilize it here?)

SCENARIO 1 – "THE KITCHEN SINK" CLIENT

This client comes in with an entire list of things going on. Goal is to drop weight and get out of the chronic pain and discomfort, regain energy, and increase hormonal balance!

- 100 lbs + Overweight
- Mid 40s
- Injuries to both shoulders and ankles; low back and cervical discs either bulging or herniated
- Fairly flexible and has good athletic acumen
- Tends to overdo training and then hurt after (which isn't good for the goal of dropping the fat)
- Thinks he knows everything; questions everything you know
- Has hormone imbalances, chronic fatigue and body aches, constant inflammation

What else do you need to know in order to start? What questions will you ask of the client?

What kind of plan are you thinking about putting the client on? 3 – 6 – 9 – 12-month plan?

SCENARIO 2 – "READY TO GO RAH RAH CRASH" CLIENT

This client comes to you rip roaring to go - usually before a family get together, wedding, or event that they have to look good for, or New Year, Spring Clean, and Bikini Beach Summer, etc.

- 20-30 lbs. overweight
- Late 20s early 30s
- No real injuries except that pesky neck and back issue from a car accident 10 years ago
- High GET STARTED motivation with no real LONG TERM stick-to-it-ness
- Tends to start and stop a lot and gets distracted by every new fad diet, pill, get fit quick program
- YO YO to the end!

What will you do with this client to make sure that the program is stuck to?

How will you motivate and educate this client so that the work you do will last a lifetime instead of the length of the next commercial fad that comes around?

____

____

____

____

____

SCENARIO 3 – "THE MEDICAL REFERRAL" CLIENT

This client has diabetes and a low level thyroid condition. Doctor has referred patient to you to create an 8-week plan to reduce blood sugar levels and save foot and leg from amputation.

- 60 lbs overweight
- Legs are fairly severe due to diabetes and would like to save from amputation
- This person let themselves go to the brink before seeking help and has NO knowledge of proper health nutrition or exercise (starting from scratch)
- Mid 40s, smoker most of life but wants to quit
- Trouble walking because of feet

What medical history questions will you need to ask the prescribing doctor?

____

____

____

____

____

What exercises may be contraindicated and what exercises will be absolutely critical?

How much mindset work will be needed and in what way will you help this client both be motivated to work with you, but also have hope that what you are doing will work?

DISCUSSION & NOTES:

THIS IS WHERE YOU WILL DESIGN YOUR PROGRAMS

DISCUSSION & NOTES:

THIS IS WHERE YOU WILL DESIGN YOUR PROGRAMS

LEVEL II: MODULE III

INTRODUCTION TO CREATING THE MINDSET OF CHANGE

MODULE III:

INTRODUCTION TO CREATING THE MINDSET OF CHANGE

TRAINING ON HOW TO ENSURE YOUR CLIENTS MAINTAIN LONG-TERM RESULTS

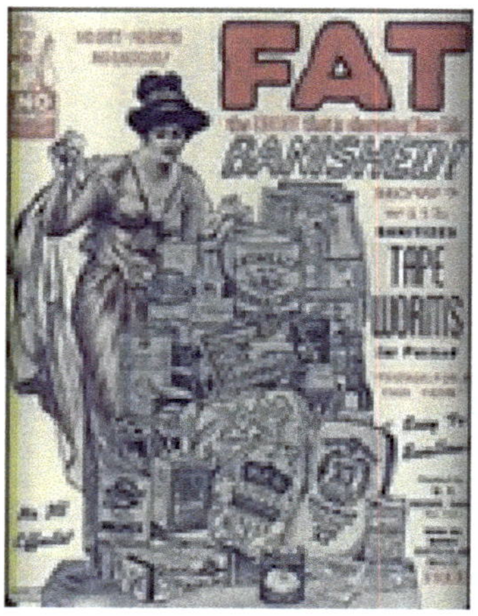

**How often do you hear the questions,
"Is this covered by my insurance?"
or "Will I have to change EVERYTHING in my life?"
"Will I still be able to have ANY fun or live a NORMAL life?"**

Our society has programmed people into believing in and wanting a magical pill or miracle cure that will take all of their pain away and give them a healthy body. Advertisers love to tout the newest super-food or pill that will help you lose weight and feel great without a change to your lifestyle.

This advertisement is a perfect example. Just eat sanitized tape worms and lose weight with no diet or exercise.

In medical terms it is as simple as "take this medication and weight will fall off," or "inflammation and pain will go away." The only caveat is that you have to take them for the rest of your life and they have a slew of side effects.

SO HOW DO WE "CREATE THE MINDSET OF CHANGE"?

First of all, we need to know that this is a problem. We need to recognize it and address it with clients directly and at the beginning of working with them. Education about this mindset is important in opening the dialogue and addressing the concerns that people have. It is not simply enough to answer the questions they have without the education about WHY it is important to work towards shifting the mindset.

"People are programmed NOT to Change!" "WHAT?" you say. Yes, people are programmed not to change."

Ari Gronich, The Performance Therapist

INTERACTIVE DRILL

Perhaps you have had a client who listened to everything you taught them, got great results, and a year later came back having reverted to the old pathologies. However, in many cases, they even came back to you worse than when they first came to you for help.

Have you thought about how to end that cycle? If yes, in what way do you plan to achieve that?

____

____

____

____

____

What are the ways in which you have led your clients to make long-term lifestyle shifts?

____

____

____

____

____

According to statistics, we are becoming more and more ill as a population while we are spending more and more money on health. So the question that begs to be answered is, "What is the cause of the results we are seeing?" Our answer is: it is our mindset.

We are being programmed by the food we consume, the television we watch, the news we hear, and the advertisements that we see. We are made to KNOW, without a shadow of a doubt, that we are getting sicker and there is nothing that will cure us...except for the latest miracle cure being advertised.

We have treatments for everything if you stick to them for the rest of your life, but there is no cure. We are told that medicine treats disease and that food and lifestyle alone cannot treat nor cure. In fact, if a doctor or health professional or company were to tell you that certain foods are equivalent in medicinal value to certain medicines, that person might be discredited by traditional or other less enlightened medical colleagues.

We all have witnessed people who have been fined, arrested, investigated, and have had their professional credentials taken, so always be cognizant of what you say and how you say it.

Even those of us in the industry have trouble understanding the overwhelming amount of information that people are being bombarded with on a regular basis. Combine strategic misinformation with a society that operates on an instant gratification lifestyle, with the 77,000+ environmental toxins that effect and affect everything from energy and pain signaling to neurological and chemical function of our bodies, and we have created a cycle that perpetuates the mindset of illness and disease.

We are a society of instant gratification, crash diets, lose 10 lbs. in 10 days, take this one pill and watch as your fat melts and all your sickness and pain vanish. Just never ever stop taking the one pill, never stop doing the one exercise, never stop, never stop, and never stop. Until the next fad or trick comes out.

So how do we, as a society of health professionals, help create a shift away from this mindset?

"We must create a society of highly-trained professionals who make it their mission to usher in a new way of thinking and doing. It takes courageous magnetic leaders to push against the status quo and move people towards a transformation of mind."

Ari Gronich, The Performance Therapist

DETOX

We have found that beginning any healing modality with a great detoxifying cleanse will initiate a cycle of health that most clients have never experienced before. This includes allowing brain function and the body's chemistry to begin the process of stimulating new neuropathways that allow for a higher level of critical thinking.

If clients are being educated while they experience this chemical change, you are creating a patterned result which is equivalent to teaching someone to fish rather than simply fishing for them.

Every emotional response to stimulus is dictated by a complex series of chemical reactions that stem from hormonal and neural communication. When a client's hormonal system is toxic and imbalanced, so too become their reasoning and actions. People are literally programmed for specific responses, and it is not until we alter their chemistry in significant and permanent ways do we achieve re-patterning of highly embedded responses.

What most people don't realize, even in the health arena, is that the majority of hormonal reactions take place not in the coinciding organs, such as Thyroid Gland producing T3 and T4, but in the gut which, when working properly, is responsible for much of our hormonal balance. We will get more deeply entrenched in this in the advanced classes; however, knowing the importance of proper gut health for hormonal balances is important when thinking about all the roles our hormones play - including how we think and our associated emotions.

As we begin to balance our body's chemistry through powerful detoxification protocols, we can now have a deep effect not only on the overall health of our clients but also on the degree to which they stick to the lifestyle changes we are making in their lives. Mindset is altered because chemistry is balanced; therefore, decision making, emotional responses, and lifestyle patterns are balanced.

Do you offer your current clients a detoxification protocol? If so, which one and why have you decided on it?

We have included a sample functional medicine grade detoxification program in Appendix A for you to begin implementing with your clients.

EASTERN VS. WESTERN MEDICINE

The goal here is to change paradigms. We no longer want to have a mindset of solely going to a medical doctor and taking medicines to heal.

The charts below are a great place to express this philosophy to a client. They give a basic understanding that is easy for them to follow and agree to.

As we look at this chart, it gives a visual example of the differences in how our two largest population societies think. It would be great if the two hands were clasped together rather than being separated because both philosophies function to provide a holistic view of the human condition.

Western vs. Eastern
Perspectives on Disease

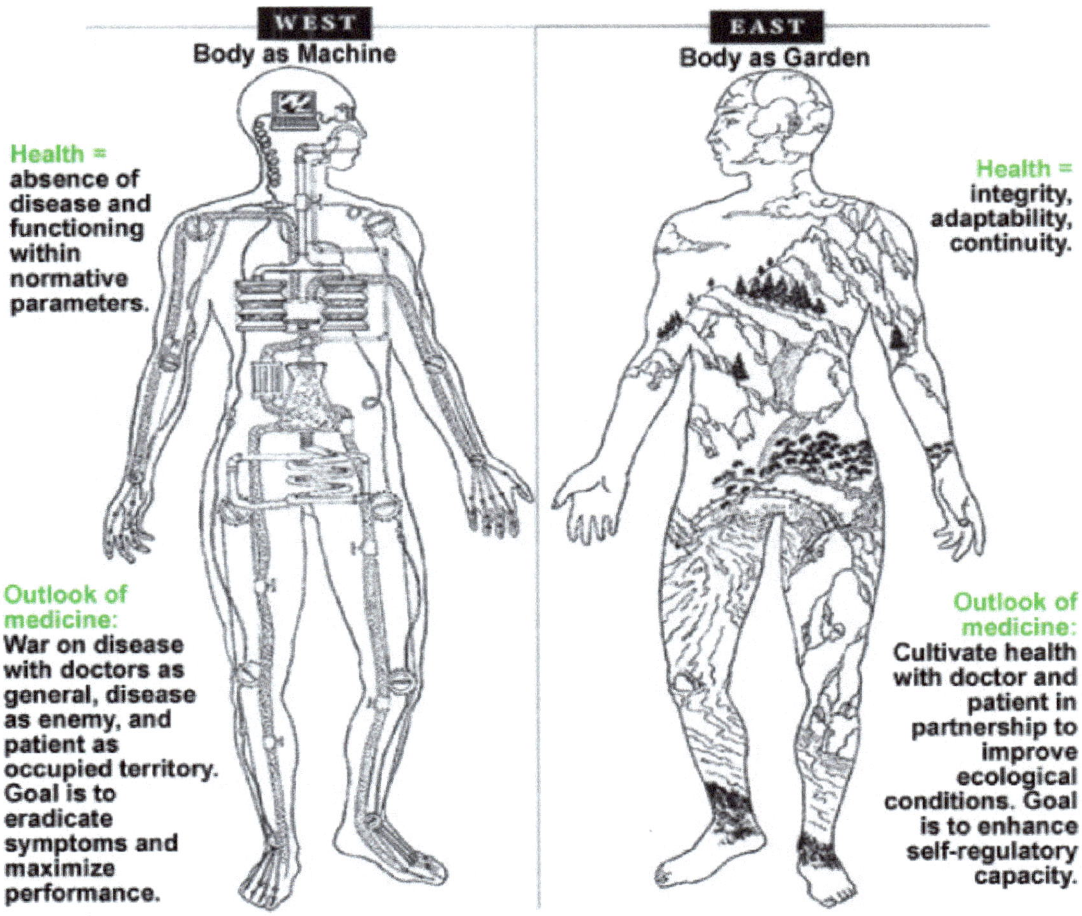

TWO MAIN SCHOOLS OF THOUGHT IN MEDICINE©

WESTERN MEDICINE	ALL FORMS OF ALTERNATIVE MEDICINE
Emergency	Preventative
Pharmaceutical	Herbal & Supplemental
Surgical	Non Invasive
Disease Oriented	Curative and Prevention of Disease
Treating Disease (Alleviates Symptoms)	Making Money While Eliminating the Problem
Making Money While Perpetuating Problem (and creating new ones)	Must Pay Attention to Your Body and create a LIFESTYLE Structured around Health and Wellness
Nothing Put in Place to Encourage Health or Disease Prevention	Grow Old Gracefully in Great Health Enjoying ALL Years of Life
Eventually Forced by Circumstances into a Life Filled with Medication, Side Effects, and Body Deterioration	Backed by thousands of years of healing legacy and is community motivated
Backed by BIG Business and is Money Motivated	OVERWHELMED AND SUPPRESSED BY WESTERN MEDICINE AND BIG BUSINESS TO THE DETRIMENT OF THE SOCIETY AND THEIR POCKETBOOKS
Now also controlled by FDA and AMA and FARMS and FOOD MANUFACTURERS putting all the CHEMICALS in our FOOD AND WATER	

Emergency and Western Medicine have a substantial role to play in our society and we would not want to dismiss it as entirely evil or negative. From the wounded on the battlefields of war to the heart attack or car accident victims that get saved, we have amazing technology and techniques that save lives.

We simply have to understand that it is not designed to create healthy lifestyles. Western medicine is not designed to keep you healthy; it is designed to help you when you are sick.

The mindset that Western societies have been pushing since the early 1900's, really since the beginning of the industrial age, has been based on remedies to problems rather than prevention of problems. As technology has shifted so that we no longer need to be out in the sun doing manual labor as much as we used to, illness and disease have risen. You would think that with the immense amount of nutrition that is available to us these days, we would all be very healthy.

Go to any grocery store and you will see a variety of colorful fruit and vegetables. THE REAL FAST FOOD...So why then is the biggest profit center of a grocery store the middle aisles with highly processed ready-to-eat meals? We live in a society that values fast and easy versus healthy and nutritious. How else can you explain the chemicals in our food? Just look at the ingredient list for a loaf of bread, and then go online and look at the ingredient list for a loaf of bread that you freshly bake at home. There is a big difference.

INTERACTIVE DISCUSSION

Which school of thought do you belong to ordinarily? Western Medicine or Alternative Medicine or both and why?

How can taking an integrative view mesh to provide greater outcomes and results for our clients?

SO WHAT DOES CAUSE CHANGES IN BEHAVIORS?

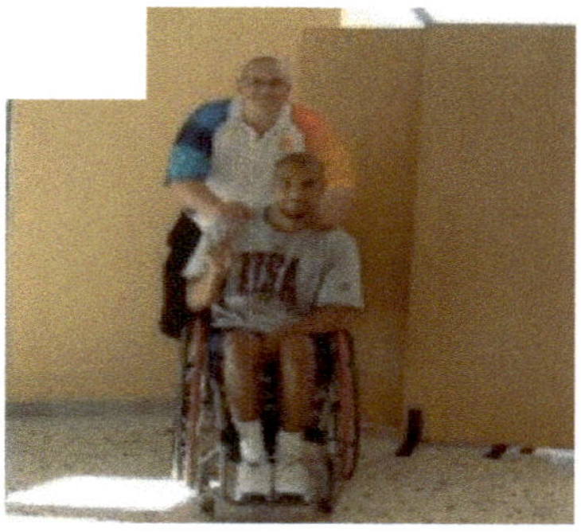

Severe pain can be so overwhelming it creates a shift that has to occur.

This is what Ari calls "**The Heal or Die Method of Change.**" An example is the drunk driver who gets in a head-on collision, his life passes in front of his eyes, and in that instant, he is completely sobered up for good.

Extreme Pleasure and Satisfaction – Something so unexpectedly wonderful occurs that your old paradigm has shifted forever. The playboy who falls in love and his old ways are finally over.

WHY DO MOST PEOPLE FAIL OR GIVE UP?

The shift happens too slowly or too subtly for people to notice, OR the pleasure from the change plateaus and ceases to provide the high it once gave. This is the **"what have you done for me lately?"** mindset. Also, this relates to the amount of knowledge you can bestow on someone. If you educate your clients WHILE simultaneously giving them the experience of change, they are more likely to continue on the path, rather than just giving them the experience or just lecturing the information.

Peer pressure and environmental stressors play a role; however, not as much as you think. How difficult is it to get a hard core vegan to eat a steak?

Why is the pain of seeing so many of our friends, relatives, and loved ones dying of Cancer, Heart Disease, Obesity, Diabetes, Chronic Pain, and Stress NOT enough to get the mind to shift? Sometimes it is. Sometimes it sends us deeper down the rabbit hole!

DISCUSSION:

How do we get someone to experience all of these life changes in a way that forces the paradigm shift into them?

Where does chemistry play a role, and how fast can we get someone's brain chemistry to shift so that they can also experience a deep enough shift of experience to cause them to continue on a path of health and vitality and extreme performance?

Do you test your clients for brain chemistry? If not, would you like to know how it can benefit your practice and separate you from the competition?

TURNING YOU INTO A RESULTS-ORIENTED PERFORMANCE THERAPIST

WHAT DO YOU DO WHEN YOU HAVE A CLIENT COME IN WHO IS NOT GETTING RESULTS?

- **Do you keep the client anyway as long as they pay?**
- **Do you fire the client and send them on their merry way?**
- **Do you refer the client to another professional?**
- **Do you collaborate with other practitioners? Which ones?**
- **What are other options?**

So how do we change the way a society was brought up to think?

What has to happen in the mind to create permanent change?

In order to alter the mindset, you have to identify what the current mindset is, and educate people on an alternative. Rather than bash the current mindset, let's replace it with a more productive one. This will be a great step in keeping your clients on track to obtain results instead of the yoyo effect that plagues so many of us.

ALTERING THE MINDSET OF WESTERN MEDICINAL THINKING

INJURY REHAB & RELAXATION/LUXURY

- Costs Rise with Age
- Emergency
- Pain Management
- Stress Management
- Always Recovering from Something
- Therapy Focused on Specific Injury
- Fixing/Making Better
- Medication/Side Effects
- Stops, Alters, or Adversely Affects "How" you are
- Pain, Misery, Stress, Disease, Tiredness, etc.

WELLNESS/PREVENTATIVE & PERFORMANCE ENHANCEMENT TRAINING

- Costs Decrease with Age
- Becomes Your Lifestyle/Part of Who You Are
- Pain Prevention
- Stress Prevention
- Injury Prevention
- Focused Training/General Fitness and Wellness
- Necessary to Maintain Health Throughout Your Life
- Takes a Few Hours a Few Times a Week
- Live Longer, Happier, and Healthier

What would you do if you had a client who was not getting results?

What is the action you agree to take immediately if a client is not obtaining success? How do you take responsibility for the results of your clients?

RESULTS GAINED EQUATE TO YOUR PROFESSIONAL IMAGE

By developing a strategy and having an oath with yourself to be 100% results oriented and not step out of your professional boundaries, you will gain great respect in both the fitness and therapy industries.

THE PERFORMANCE THERAPIST SUCCESS EXAMPLE

WHAT WILL BE YOUR IMPACT ON YOUR CLIENTS?

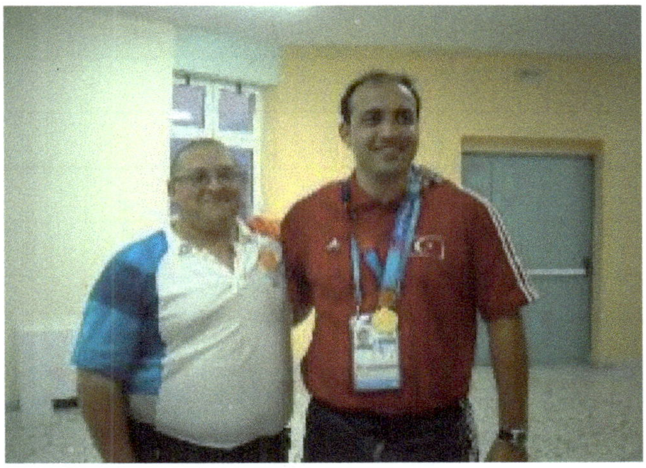

Example:

This Paralympic athlete from Turkey in Athens during the 2004 games had no leg and was competing in both indoor and outdoor shooting. We worked on mindset, focus, and visualizing the results he wanted. The next day, he came back and put that gold medal around my neck after having broken almost every Olympic, Paralympic, and World Record in his sport. THE POWER OF MINDSET.

What are some solutions that can work for you to expedite the mindset shift in your clients? Most people come to you because they WANT to change. They simply don't know how. They don't have the education, skills, tools, and especially, the mindset. Let's give you some tools that have worked for many.

DISCUSSION:

What is your Why? (What drives you? What brought you into this industry?)

What is the impact that you would like to leave on your clients?

What is the impact you would like to leave on the industry?

NOTES:

THE BASICS AND POWER OF MEDITATION

Educating Your Clients on the Physical and Neurological Benefits of Regular Meditation

HERE ARE SOME STATISTICS FROM THE AMERICAN PSYCHOLOGICAL ASSOCIATION AS OF 2015:

Statistic Verification	
Source: American Psychological Association, American Institute of Stress, NY	
Research Date: 7.8.2014	

Top Causes of Stress in the U.S.

	Cause	Factors
1	Job Pressure	Co-Worker Tension, Bosses, Work Overload
2	Money	Loss of Job, Reduced Retirement, Medical Expenses
3	Health	Health Crisis, Terminal or Chronic Illness
4	Relationships	Divorce, Death of Spouse, Arguments with Friends, Loneliness
5	Poor Nutrition	Inadequate Nutrition, Caffeine, Processed Foods, Refined Sugars
6	Media Overload	Television, Radio, Internet, E-Mail, Social Networking
7	Sleep Deprivation	Inability to release adrenaline and other stress hormones

U.S Stress Statistics	**Data**
Percent of people who regularly experience physical symptoms caused by stress	77 %
Regularly experience psychological symptoms caused by stress	73 %
Feel they are living with extreme stress	33 %
Feel their stress has increased over the past five years	48 %
Cited money and work as the leading cause of their stress	76 %
Reported lying awake at night due to stress	48 %
Stress Impact Statistics	
Percent who say stress has a negative impact on their personal and professional life	48 %
Employed adults who say they have difficulty managing work and family responsibilities.	31 %
Percent who cited jobs interfering with their family or personal time as a significant source of stress.	35 %
Percent who said stress has caused them to fight with people close to them	54 %
Reported being alienated from a friend or family member because of stress	26 %
Annual costs to employers in stress related health care and missed work.	$300 Billion
Percent who say they are "always" or "often" under stress at work	30 %
People who cited physical symptoms experienced the following	
Fatigue	51 %
Headache	44 %
Upset stomach	34 %
Muscle tension	30 %
Change in appetite	23 %
Teeth grinding	17 %
Change in sex drive	15 %
Feeling dizzy	13 %
People who cited psychological symptoms experienced the following	
Irritability or anger	50 %
Feeling nervous	45 %
Lack of energy	45 %
Feeling as though you could cry	35 %

STRESS IS THE LEADING CAUSE OF DISEASE IN AMERICA TODAY - WE NEED WAYS TO BEAT IT.

> *"If stress is the biggest cause of disease, then it is intrinsically important for any health and fitness professional to gain expertise in relaxation and meditative techniques."*
>
> **Ari Gronich, The Performance Therapist**

What do you do in order to bring relaxation and meditation into your life? How do you unwind?

Without a productive way to release stress, anxiety, and tension, we bottle up these emotions until they have a profound impact on our health and overall wellbeing. Cortisol, our stress hormone, is one of the major causes of belly fat and a sign that your adrenal system is overloaded. This causes your body to constantly be in a state of fight or flight which draws vital nutrients and blood supply and oxygen away from your organs and pools them into your extremities. This overload is great if you are about to be attacked by a lion in the jungle, but for general living purposes, it makes it difficult for your body to be able to recover from illness and disease.

A SIMPLE DEFINITION OF MEDITATION: "THE ACT OR PROCESS OF SPENDING TIME IN QUIET THOUGHT" – MERRIAM-WEBSTER

Meditation comes in many forms. It could be 10 minutes in the morning breathing deeply while slowly getting ready for the day. It could be guided meditation, which has been shown to be great at preparing someone for a job interview, sporting competition, or even before a first date. Meditation can be done solely or in groups.

Methods and beliefs around meditation vary from culture to culture. Zen meditation is the silent, non-moving variety of meditation in which one or a group sits in silence allowing all thought to pass through without judgment. With walking meditation, as you move you become aware not only of your thoughts but the feeling of movement in your body and how those sensations are interlinked with thought.

Listening to Binaural and Isochronic tones at different frequencies can be extremely beneficial to your clients both during workout as well as meditation. You can find on YouTube hundreds of different patterns and tones and frequencies designed to alter your brain chemistry and brain states. From alpha to delta to beta and theta, each state creates a different biological reaction in your body and these can be a great addition to your meditation experience.

In western culture, meditation could be anything from staring at a candle to fishing on the water, to zoning out in the kitchen cooking.

Popular amongst many celebrities these days is Transcendental Meditation, a Hindu modality in which a person is looking to achieve a relaxed state through regular periods of chanting a mantra of some kind.

Whichever method of meditation you choose, the science is in, and meditation does alter brain chemistry and physical neurology.

BENEFITS OF MEDITATION INCLUDE:

- Deeper ability to concentrate on tasks
- Lower blood pressure and resting heart rate
- A reduction in depression and anxiety as well as overall psychological well-being
- According to Functional MRI's, meditation seems to have a range of neurological benefits – from alterations in grey matter volume to a reduction in activity in the "me" centers of the brain, to enhanced connections between different regions of the brain.

Sara Lazar and her team at Harvard found that mindfulness meditation can actually change the structure of the brain: Eight weeks of Mindfulness-Based Stress Reduction (MBSR) was found to increase cortical thickness in the hippocampus, which governs learning and memory, and in certain areas of the brain that play roles in emotion regulation and self-referential processing. There were also decreases in brain cell volume in the amygdala, which is responsible for fear, anxiety, and stress – and these changes matched the participants' self-reports of their stress levels, indicating that meditation not only changes the brain, but it changes our subjective perception and feelings as well.

In fact, a follow-up study by Lazar's team found that after meditation training, changes in brain areas linked to mood and arousal were also linked to improvements in how participants said they felt - i.e., their psychological well-being. So for anyone who says that activated blobs in the brain don't necessarily mean anything, our subjective experience – improved mood and well-being – does indeed seem to be shifted through meditation as well.

Study Source:
http://www.ncbi.nlm.nih.gov/pmc/articles/PMC3004979/

ArticleSource:
http://www.forbes.com/sites/alicegwalton/2015/02/09/7-ways-meditation-can-actually-change-the-brain/#6ba4005b7023

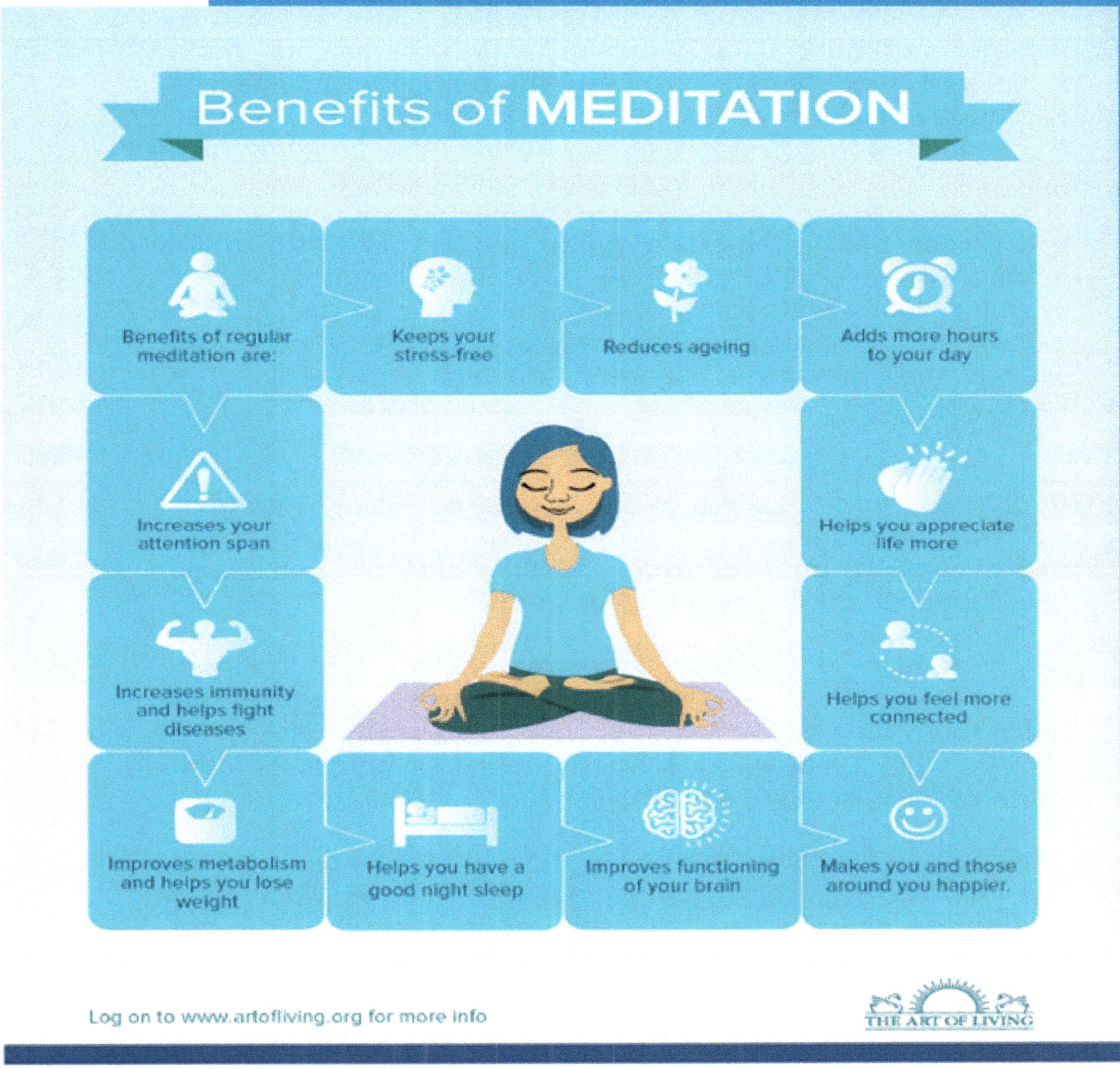
Benefits of MEDITATION
Benefits of regular meditation are:
Keeps your stress-free
Reduces ageing
Adds more hours to your day
Helps you appreciate life more
Helps you feel more connected
Makes you and those around you happier.
Improves functioning of your brain
Helps you have a good night sleep
Improves metabolism and helps you lose weight
Increases immunity and helps fight diseases
Increases your attention span
Log on to www.artofliving.org for more info
THE ART OF LIVING

GUIDED MEDITATION AND THE BENEFITS FOR PERFORMANCE THERAPISTS TO USE WITH THEIR CLIENTS

Guided meditation is a process by which one or more participants meditate in response to the guidance provided by a trained practitioner or teacher, either in person or via a written text, sound recording, video, or audiovisual medium comprising music or verbal instruction, or a combination of both.

As a trainer, having the skill to guide people in meditation will enhance the overall effectiveness of your programs as well as providing your clients with a deeper level of trust and faith in you. When you begin to open someone up to the subconscious levels of their brain, they inherently develop a higher level of trust in you.

For example, you have a group of diabetics who are all struggling with the exercise and eating plans. You get them all into a room together for a 15-minute guided meditation. As you begin speaking, and they begin to drift into your voice, you have them intently listening to your words.

Their heart rate begins to slow down and the voices inside them are silencing as they are listening to you. Now you begin to talk to their organs about how they are functioning beautifully, enjoying all of the new foods that are being consumed and the nutrition that is being absorbed.

They begin to relax their breathing and now you begin to talk to their joints and muscles about how good it feels when they exercise properly. You talk about the strength they are producing and how nice it feels to have good posture. You will actually see their posture straightening out.

In the above paragraph, I was gently guiding you in a meditation. You could not only hear my voice, but you could feel what was happening in your room with your clients.

How much more likely will that group of clients be to continue on the plan that you have designed for them?

A group setting can be powerful because you are developing a community amongst your clients in which they begin supporting each other as well, further increasing the results you will achieve with your clients.

Everyone responds to stimuli differently. Some people hear, some see, others are more kinesthetic and they sense and feel. When guiding a group through a meditation process, remember to use words that stimulate ALL of the senses. You will get even the most difficult people engaged in the process. Have your clients either close their eyes when guiding them through a meditation or, if you like, have them focus on a single object. A candle flame is a great object to focus on as the dancing of the flame calms the conscious brain and allows you to go deeper into the subconscious mind.

This can be very powerful if you have an athlete who is getting ready to compete. We always recommend to our professional athlete clients that they do not practice the day before a big competition. That should be a day they take to relax and meditate about the competition. It is almost like day-dreaming although, if they have a great specialist like yourselves, having a guided meditation is ideal. You guide them through every movement, every sound, and every moment of the competition. It has been scientifically proven that when you are visualizing, your muscles twitch the same as they do if you are actually physically doing the movement. You activate the same parts of the brain that are active, and you actually put into muscle cell memory those movements.

The more you visualize and meditate on what goals you want to achieve, the more your brain recognizes that as your natural state - thus altering the neuropathways that lead to a change in habits and behaviors. This is where that saying "Mind over Matter" comes into play.

There are internal and external types of imagery and visualization you can utilize when guiding clients. Internal imagery is when your clients are placing themselves in the action you are describing. They are the athlete; they feel it in their bones. External imagery is third person where you are guiding them in a way that they are watching the action as though it is on a movie screen and they are the audience of the show. Both of these techniques have their place. It can take pressure off the person if what they are hearing is an observation rather than a personal action. External imagery can alleviate the anxiety that many people feel as patterns of thought get adjusted; being the person in the show, internal imagery, is great for building up the neuropathways.

Imagine the difference between playing football in the Super Bowl and watching it on the screen with some buddies. Watching, you can get to a place where you feel it; however, it is not the same as being IN it. So our recommendation is to develop a guided meditation that includes both points of view. For creating real changes, internal imagery has been shown to be more effective than external imagery.

CHAMPION GOLFER JACK NICKLAUS SAID,

"I never hit a shot, not even in practice, without having a very sharp, in-focus picture of it in my head. First I see the ball where I want it to finish, nice and white and sitting up high on the bright green grass. Then the scene quickly changes, and I see the ball going there; its path, trajectory, and shape, even its behavior on landing."

DISCUSSION:

Provide several specific ways that you will implement this in your practice.

How will you be able to measure the success of implementing this?

Is meditation or guided imagery a substitute for action?

INTERACTIVE DRILL

CREATING A POWERFUL PERFORMANCE THERAPIST PRACTICE

SAMPLE MEDITATION

Everyone reacts differently to various stimuli. This meditation is designed to target all listening styles for maximum efficacy:

Imagine for a moment that you are sitting down in your favorite chair. This chair could be anywhere in your house, your work, or even in a kayak. The only requisite is that the chair is your favorite, most comfortable place to sit. It is where you relax the deepest.

This chair molds to your body engulfing you into the most comfortable supported posture you could possibly imagine. As you sit in this chair, you begin to drift off a little bit.

You are starting to daydream and envision what your life is like. You can see, hear, taste, smell, and touch all that you have created. You are a successful business person. You have hundreds and thousands of positive, raving fans giving their testimonials about the results you have delivered. You have changed the lives of those who suffered pain and illness.

As you look back from this place of ultimate success and ultimate satisfaction in what you have accomplished and who you are, you begin to drift deeper into your imagination. You begin to breathe more slowly and with more deliberation. Your body is beginning to tingle and feel alive with oxygen.

You take this journey back step by step, and you are looking at this much like a home video you once made. If you are old enough, you may remember the reel to reel or VHS tapes and the quality of videotaping. The imperfections of the video only add texture and character, allowing you to feel deeply the life you have led.

You can smell the smells, and taste the tastes, feel the feels, and hear the sounds. You are remembering the beginning. How hard it was getting started. The blood, sweat, and tears that you put into building your business. You experience the classes and learning of the material all over again - remembering all of the critical information that would get you to pass your test. You remember leaving school so proud of your accomplishment and passionate about your choice to live this life.

You can feel how determined you are to make a difference and change people's lives for the better. You are deeply grateful and scared about how you are going to make it all work.

And as you look back from this viewing room, watching your life on the screen, you notice how rhythmic your breath is, and the tempo of your slowly-beating heart. You notice how relaxed your muscles have become and how they change tonality through the different stages of your life. You drift deeper into a state of maximum relaxation and satisfaction.

You can see the moment you got your very first customer; the first person to walk into your doors and sign up. You can see the first 10 clients who did it all together in your first group class. How beautiful and inspiring it was to see them all support each other while pushing through the ups and downs and pain and tiredness and stubbornness. Feel every emotion you went through fighting to keep your dreams alive - the joy when you had someone who said, "Let me help you."

You can see every failure that you turned into a success and every success that catapulted you to the next level. You can even remember and watch that first day you worked with your business coach and wrote your first business plan, marketing plan, vision statement, and more. You remember the first client that you fired because you just weren't a fit to work with each other, and you drift by that moment when you knew from the depths of your soul that you were in JUST THE RIGHT PLACE.

You pass by the miracles that were created at your hands, head, and heart, and you fly by the times when nothing seemed to work out.

Now you are in full-fledged success mode. You have passed through the test and it is time for even more growth. It is time to take on employees and adopt new policies and get more education. It is time to expand and help more and more people. You taste the dinner that you had with your first new employee on the day your expectations were exceeded and you just had to celebrate.

Remember the comfortable chair you are sitting in. How relaxed your muscles are and how your aches and pains just vanish. See yourself working less now, and earning more money. You have created amazing training systems and delegated tasks to others so that you can enjoy the fruits of your labor more.

You have developed your own economy and are not only supporting the health of your clients but also the lives of your employees and contractors. You have a philosophy that breeds loyalty and hard work with heart and purpose. You have created online programs that feed you more clients and support your ever-growing reach as you touch more and more lives, while living a relaxed lifestyle that supports your many hobbies and interests. The world is impacted by all of the work that you have done and accomplished.

As you begin to make your way closer and closer to the present, you are getting more and more energized. You bless the time that you have spent studying your past and remembering every detail and aspect of becoming this highly-productive successful medical fitness professional. You laugh a little reminiscing of all of the people you touched and watching the stories of them unfold.

You are getting more and more energized now, as your muscles begin to twitch and you experience the feeling of coming back into your present body. You remember everything that you saw; your future as you would like it to be can unfold before you, and you FEEL that PASSION flooding into your body.

Ready to learn more. Ready to grow deeper.

You will come back into your body refreshed and relaxed and rejuvenated. You will remember everything that happened in your future. The timeline is your creating and you can come back to this meditation anytime you want, to shift directions into your chosen future.

You can begin to open your eyes, knowing that you can give to your clients the experience you just had - adapting it specifically for them, to help ease stress and to support great overall health.

That passion you have is fully alive in you as you awaken.

HAVE CLIENTS GET UP AND MOVE, AND GET THE FEELING BACK INTO THEIR BODIES!

INTERACTIVE BUSINESS - BUILDING DRILL BONUS

TO SUPPORT YOUR PERFORMANCE THERAPY BUSINESS

BUSINESS VISION BOARDS

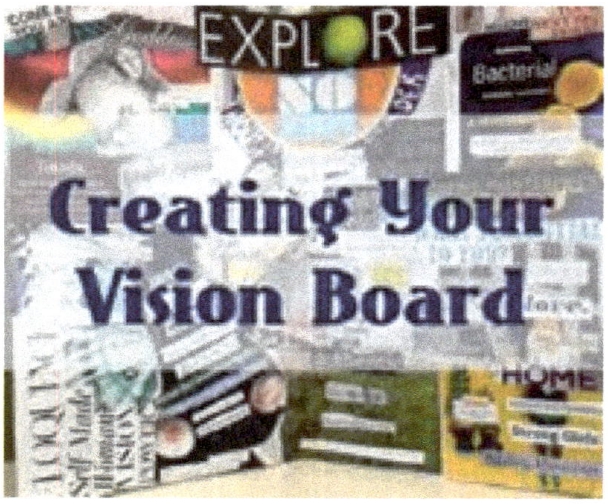

As an added benefit to your clients, as well as a possible revenue-generating activity, have a group vision board day where everyone gets together to create their personal vision boards. You can charge $25 - $50 per person. If you have 10 clients in the class, you just made an extra $500 while providing your clients added benefit and a sense of community. This is a great way to separate yourself from others in your field. Ask yourself the following questions to grow your business; see the paragraph below for ideas to help your clients with their vision boards.

HOW MUCH MONEY DO YOU WANT TO MAKE?

WHAT IS YOUR IDEAL CLIENT? WHOM DO YOU LOVE TO WORK WITH?

WHAT DOES THE BUILDING LOOK LIKE THAT YOU ARE WORKING IN?

WHAT LOCATION IN THE WORLD DO YOU WANT TO WORK IN?

WHAT OUTCOMES DO YOU WANT FOR YOUR CLIENTS?

If you do not have a vision board day or afternoon for your clients, have them create a vision board at home of who they want to be and what they want to have in their life. This includes what they want to look like and how they want to feel. It should include foods they love eating and some that they are addicted to that they want to change. Create a poster-board-sized vision board that is large enough for them to see it. If you own your own studio or have a large enough office, you may want to put them up so that as you are working with your clients, everyone can see regularly what they want to accomplish, but also root for the other people in your practice. This creates a group mentality that can socially overwhelm the societal mentality in the real world. However,

you must get permission to publicly display their information.

If they leave the vision board at home, they can see it regularly to constantly remind themselves of the progress they want to make. One important note here: engage any family members and friends of importance to the client in the process. It is a vicious uphill battle that very rarely works without their support. When I take on a new client, I always have them bring their spouse in for the consultation. This way they are aware and agreeing to be on board with the transformation that is about to take place with their loved ones. This is crucial to long-term success.

ACTION PLAN

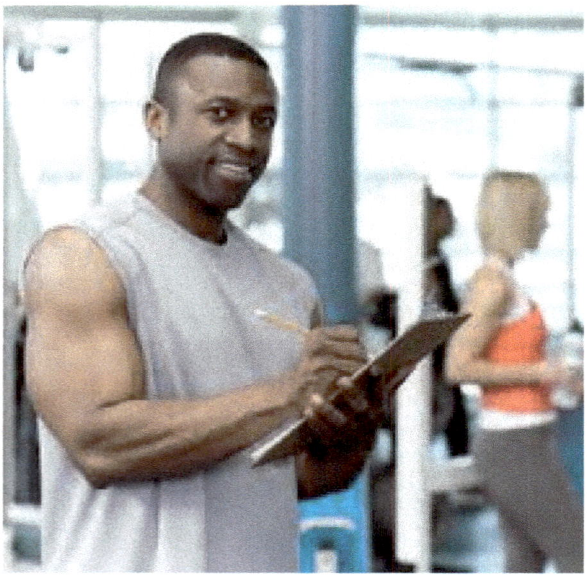

Congratulations!

Remember, we said that we need to change the mindset of our clients to achieve real change. Education is the beginning of that process. Engaging people in a process that both educates them and shows them results is even better. When we can engage people in a physical experience or proof positive of a concept, then we can obtain real change.

**"Tell me, and I may remember.
Show me, and I will remember.
Involve me, and I will understand."
Chinese Proverb**

As you take your clients through the process of experiencing health, educating them as to what you are doing, why it is working, what the mechanisms of action are having on them, and how the continued action will create lifelong results, you will increase your percentage of clients who live these healthy lifestyles for the rest of their lives.

WORKSHOP CONCLUSION

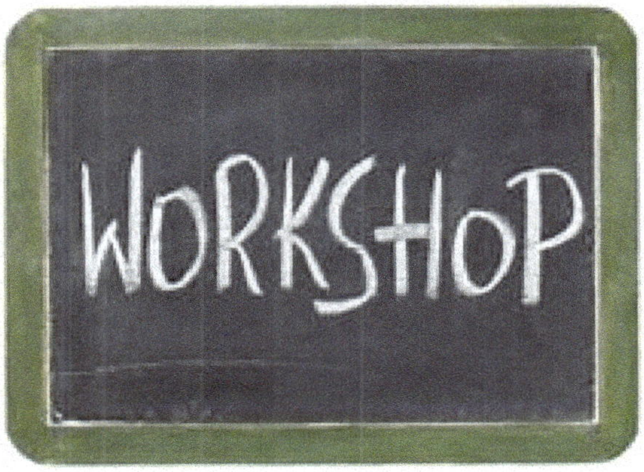

You have just finished two days with us. We have barely broken the surface of what there is to know, learn, and master. Continuing your education with each successive workshop system we offer will take you to ever-expanding results. It is also very important that you start implementing the principles you've learned, because knowledge without practice is like a hammer in a drawer. The tools only work when used.

""The beginning of learning any good methodology is developing a foundation from which all things can grow."

Ari Gronich, The Performance Therapist

In this level we touched on the power of a world-class evaluation process that assesses the needs of patients who have been referred to you by other medical professionals. Not only does this increase the quality of results you receive, but it also drives your professionalism and highlights that you are a specialist with a unique set of expertise.

We were also able to experiment with exercises that are unusual, yet very powerful, for obtaining tremendous gains in a wide range of motion, flexibility, power, strength, and speed. These exercises have the added benefit of developing a highly injury-resistant body.

Both as a client and a therapist, you were in the position of experiencing how to utilize our methodology and obtain a deep sense of what you are putting your clients through. This will raise your awareness and empathy, allowing you to better tailor your treatment to your clients' specific needs. You will know what they are experiencing so you can tweak and shift exercises with ease, giving them deeper and more effective results.

We learned about mindset and how important the approach we take is with regards to the quality of our outcomes. If we shift our own mindset and learn to shift the mindset of our clients, we can truly create a healthier, more joyful, and active society. We will stem the tide of disease and illness, returning a higher quality of life to everyone.

Take this knowledge and implement the principles of this methodology,

Get ready for your business to expand, because now you have the skills to provide results that are second to none in your area.

END NOTES:

APPENDIX A
REFERENCE

Use the following expert leaders as reference points to provide you a complete learning experience:

Dr. Douglas Gillard, BS, DC, Spine Researcher

https://www.youtube.com/watch?v=3YnMzXOTd2I;%20www.chirogeek.com

National Electronic Injury Surveillance System

http://www.cpsc.gov/en/Research--Statistics/NEISS-Injury-Data/

Western vs Eastern Perspectives

https://www.google.com/url?sa=i&rct=j&q=&esrc=s&source=images&cd=&cad=rja&uact=8&ved=0ahUKEwi4naK5uNDNAhUHzz4KHUzdDbQQjB0IBg&url=http%3A%2F%2Fphysicalculturist.ca%2Fwestern-vs-eastern-medicine%2F&bvm=bv.125801520,d.amc&psig=AFQjCNHYBl0KdF3ULG9-KbGEQju30ltPsg&ust=1467399817805085

disclosure.pdf | consentform.pdf | Consent Form Disclosure.pdf | California Senate Bill SB-577.pdf | Lab Values Chart 120511.pdf | NerveChart.pdf | spinescan.pdf

APPENDIX B
POWER PARTNERSHIP

Attendees - Use the following educational resources to help grow your medical exercise knowledge and business.

RESOURCE NAME	EMAIL ADDRESS	INFORMATION
ACHIEVE HEALTH USA	WWW.ACHIEVEHEALTHUSA.COM	BLOG AND VIDEOS
ACHIEVE SYSTEMS	WWW.ACHIEVESYSTEMSPRO.COM	BUSINESS RESOURCES
ANOVA HEALTH	WWW.ANOVAHEALTH.COM	EXTREMELY HIGH QUALITY SUPPLEMENTS THAT ARE PRESCRIPTION STRENGTH AND GRADED
IFM – INSTITUTE FOR FUNCTIONAL MEDICINE	WWW.FUNCTIONALMEDICINE.ORG	EDUCATIONAL RESOURCE
INSURANCE COMPANY	WWW.MASSAGELIABILITYINSURANCEGROUP.COM	350 MODALITIES COVERED
BODY SITE	WWW.BODYSITE.COM/ACHIEVE	ONLINE DELIVERY SYSTEM EHR PATIENT TRACKING
MEDICAL FITNESS ASSOCIATION	WWW.MEDICALFITNESS.ORG	GLOBAL NETWORK OF MEDICALLY-INTEGRATED FITNESS FACILITIES
MEDICAL FITNESS NETWORK	WWW.MEDICALFITNESSNETWORK.ORG	EDUCATIONAL RESOURCES AND MEMBERSHIP ORGANIZATION
READING X-RAYS AND MRI	WWW.CHIROGEEK.COM	EVALUATION OF IMAGES

APPENDIX C
FORMS

These forms provide you with a turn-key business system that you may use to private label and plug into your business. Success is just a few forms away.

Consultation Enrollment Form.do
HIPAA - FORM.doc
Adult - Consultatior - History.doc
Steps for Initial Consultation.docx
10 - objections.doc
About Our Presenter BIO.docx
Patient-Introductio n.docx
Achieve Health USA Disclaimer Form.doc
Funtional Wellness Intake Form.doc
New Client Contract.docx
Initial Palpation Evaluation Form.pdf
Initial Palpation Evaluation Form.doc
Detoxification Protocol

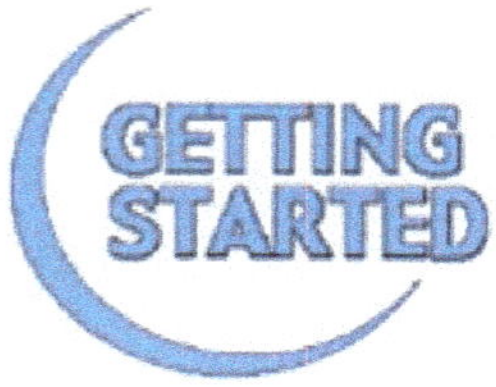

BACK-OFFICE ACCESS GRANTED

You now have full access to Performance Therapy Academy back office HUB to continue your education and on-going business and personal growth.

APPENDIX D
NOTABLE EXAMPLES

An example from Dr. Douglas Gillard

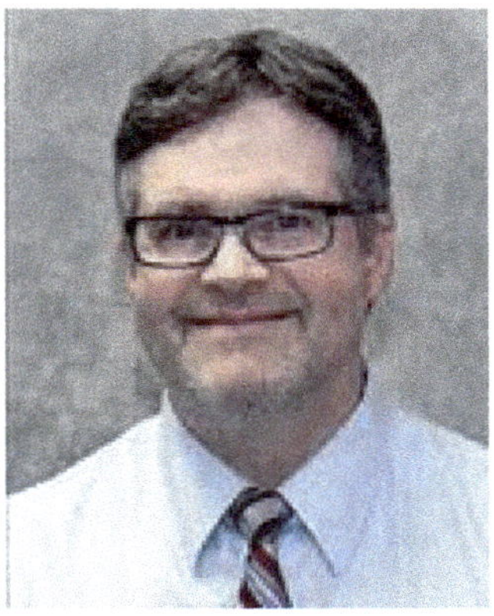

Dr. Douglas Gillard, BS, DC, Spine Researcher, has a YouTube page that offers some of the best and easiest-to-understand videos on reading MRI's. This link is to one of his videos about reading the lumbar spine: https://www.youtube.com/watch?v=3YnMzXOTd2I His website is www.chirogeek.com.

WORKSHOP EVALUATION FORM

What three key points did you learn from this workshop?

What subjects would you like more information about?

What aspects of this workshop really worked for you?

TESTIMONIAL

Name (signed):

Date:

Name (printed):

Email:

BECOME PART OF ACHIEVE ACADEMY OPTION

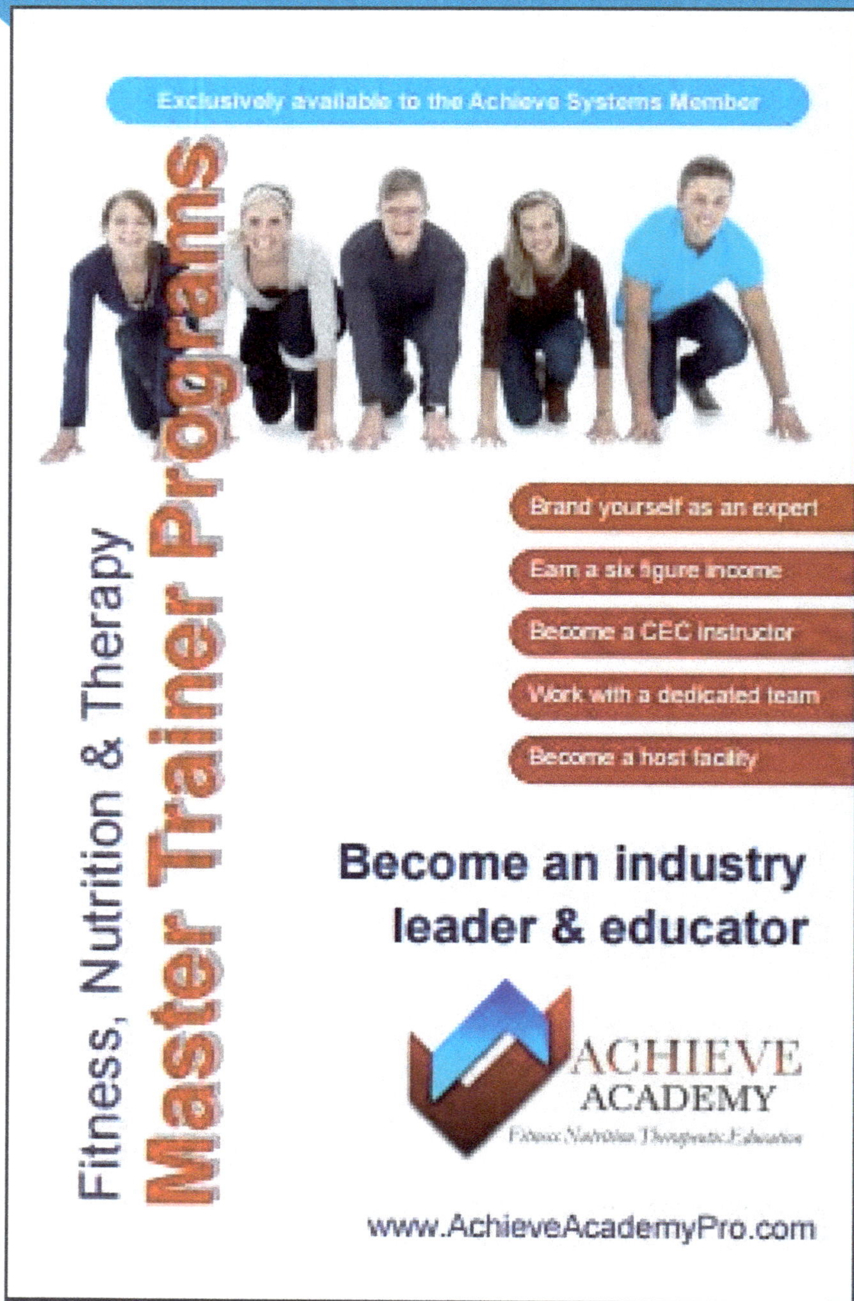

OPPORTUNITIES TO EDUCATE THE WORLD!

Must meet education requirements; please contact your Performance Therapy Academy representative for more information.

INTRODUCTION TO THE ACHIEVE SYSTEMS AND MASTER INSTRUCTOR OPPORTUNITY

Become a Master Instructor for Performance Therapy Academy

Achieve Systems is a main strategic partner with Performance Therapy Academy.

All master trainers/national-approved CEC instructors are required to be a licensee or member of Achieve Systems to ensure future success. In addition to having access to education programs like Performance Therapy Academy, you'll also be able to plug into multiple other revenue streams and coaching that will help your business thrive. Performance Therapy Academy's objective is to provide you with tools that will help you create success in your business. The strategic relationship is one of those tools.

Performance Therapy Academy is a company with decades of experience in helping fitness, nutrition, wellness, and therapy professionals acquire clients and build business, success, and wealth. We provide the top team of industry leaders and ICONS to help you grow your business. In addition, we have over 48 revenue streams that we have invested millions of dollars in, providing you with opportunities to greatly increase your bottom line with little to no investment on your part. Simply plug in, go to work, and gain huge rewards. We are all about giving you tools in your tool belt. If you are new to Achieve Systems and this opportunity, then start by putting yourself through the Discover Achieve Systems Process.

You can review details of this incredible strategic partnership at www.achievesystemspro.com.

Welcome aboard. You'll love what you see!

www.ingramcontent.com/pod-product-compliance
Lightning Source LLC
LaVergne TN
LVHW071346210926
848486LV00003B/237